The Fountain of Youth

*Autophagy Myths,
Enigmas, and the
Unaltered Truth About It*

D.R. Krauz

Table of Contents

Introduction

Since the earliest days of recorded history, humans have been searching for the mythical fountain of youth—the secret formula to reversing aging, staying healthy and vibrant, and looking our best while we're at it.

Advancements in the field of medicine have brought us multiple options, ranging from pills we can pop to surgeries, both superficial and essential. Still, the exact equation is yet to be discovered.

In the past few decades, rapid advancements in research surrounding the topic of autophagy seem to be pointing us in the right direction. Far from being a miracle cure, science is still showing a lot of promise. Mother Nature appears to have a few tricks up her sleeve that we're just now starting to understand.

We'll get into the deep science of autophagy later. Still, before you go any further reading this book, it's helpful for you to understand the basic principles of what autophagy is, how it works, and, ultimately, why we should all care.

What Is Autophagy

At its core, autophagy is the process your cells go through to recycle damaged, toxic or dead material that has accumulated inside your body due to normal biological processes and the day to day stresses of life.

Your body is equipped to capture this leftover material and convert it into energy that your healthy cells can use to continue performing their proper functions, keeping you alive and well.

When the waste is broken down into its basic components, it can also be used to repair damaged cells that may still be useful to your body.

Autophagy is the process by which all of this happens, and more.

The word autophagy derives from the Greek words "auto," meaning self, and "phagy," meaning to eat or consume.

If the thought of cannibalism makes you squeamish, you might not want to think too hard about the fact that the secret to your health and longevity might be in the hands of tiny, self-eating mechanisms inside your body.

Instead, you can think of it more like internal exfoliation. Rubbing away dead skin cells through gentle exfoliation has long been a favorite practice of many anti-aging experts.

For healthy, fresh, and clean skin to shine, you need to remove the dead skin cells as they age. Exfoliation is one way to achieve this.

You may have also seen your body's natural process of healing from sunburn. The damaged, burnt skin will separate from your new, healthy skin as it grows underneath, and eventually peel or flake off.

The cells inside your body die and are damaged just as frequently as your outer skin cells. They're just harder to see and, therefore, more often ignored.

The dead and damaged cells still need to be removed for the new, healthy cells to shine, and autophagy is your body's natural method of exfoliating and getting rid of the damage.

The best part of this system, however, isn't just the removal of damaged cells, but the recycling process. Autophagy doesn't only allow healthy young cells to excel, but it uses the waste to give them energy and to help heal and defend them when they need it.

How Does It Work

Again, we're going to go much more in-depth on this process later on in the book, but to get you started, we'll run through a simple explanation of how the process of autophagy works.

What science has been able to tell us so far is that autophagy is essentially a fail-safe protective process. When we don't provide enough new energy for our cells to survive and operate through the food we ingest, the process of autophagy is triggered.

Imagine tiny recycling units roaming around in your body, collecting anything that is either damaged or is actively damaging your body. Includes dysfunctional or dead cells, toxins that don't belong inside of us, and even some bacteria.

The recycling units collect the waste, break it all down into its most basic components - carbs, proteins, and fats - and then use those components as fuel for the cells that are lacking energy.

It's a remarkable process. Not only does autophagy clean up all the garbage that we don't want leftover in our system, but it upcycles it into something useful that helps our body function properly.

It can be challenging to wrap your mind around the concept, especially when you can't see or feel the process working for you.

Over the years, we can recognize the aging process occurring in our bodies, but on a day to day basis, we feel much the same as we did the day before. However, our cells are continually changing. New ones are created, old ones die, and damaged ones either continue to disintegrate, or they get repaired.

Just like any machine that you perform maintenance on, your body is undergoing maintenance every second of every day. Autophagy is a critical part of that process. Without it, the individual cells in our body will continue to break down through use, but not enjoy the benefits of proper maintenance.

Why Should We Care

The longer we're alive, the more stress we subject our bodies to, and the more damage gets left behind inside of us. The damage accumulates over time, and as we age, we start to see the effects more seriously.

This accumulation can lead to a variety of different age-related and metabolic diseases. If we can start to harness the power of autophagy more strategically, it logically follows that we'll be able to reduce our risk of contracting a host of different diseases.

Imagine living out your life without fear of developing Alzheimer's, diabetes, liver disease, cancer, or even superficial wrinkles.

We haven't unlocked all the answers yet, but we do know enough to potentially lower your risk for all of these diseases, while helping you maintain a healthy weight and plenty of energy, no matter what your age is.

As you work your way through this book, my goal is to provide you with enough accessible information to make you believe passionately about the power of autophagy, without any doubt.

Once you understand how it works, you'll learn how you can trigger the process in your own body to reap its many rewards. Finally, you'll be given the tools to use autophagy as proactively as possible, learning how to make lifestyle changes that will improve your quality of life in a variety of ways.

The Autophagy Lifestyle Planner

(<u>DO NOT</u> even consider inducing autophagy without it...)

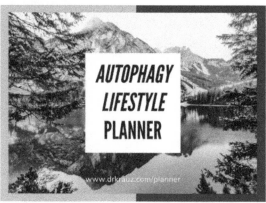

With the *Autophagy Lifestyle* Planner, you'll get:

> ➢ The **9 key elements** you cannot induce autophagy without.
>
> ➢ How to schedule them into your week, for maximum results.
>
> ➢ An effective way of keeping yourself accountable.

The last thing we want is for you to learn all the valuable information contained in this book, and not be able to put it into practice.

To receive your *Autophagy Lifestyle Planner,* visit the link: www.drkrauz.com/planner

The Fountain of Youth

D.R Krauz

Chapter 1:

Eat Your Heart Out

All human life is utterly dependent on the ability of cells to clone themselves. All organisms more complicated than a single cell have this power.

Through a process called mitosis, a single cell can divide itself into two exact duplicates. By doing so, the organism it's a part of can grow and heal.

Humans don't grow bigger because their cells grow bigger. They grow because more cells are created through this duplication process. When we injure or damage our bodies in any way, the dead and destroyed cells are eliminated, but instead of leaving a void in their place, surrounding cells divide themselves to heal the area.

Mitosis is continuously occurring in your body throughout your entire life.

Some cells, however, don't have the ability to

clone themselves. Blood cells don't have a nucleus, so they're incapable of dividing. Heart cells won't divide because they're too busy working. Once they die, they aren't replaced. Neurons, our nerve or brain cells, are incredibly complicated and specialized, and they lack a centriole, which is necessary for cell division, so they also can't clone themselves.

Yet, somehow, these cells are still able to repair themselves.

That's where autophagy and cellular recycling come into play.

Nobel Prize Worthy Research

In the grand scheme of the world of medical science, what we know about autophagy is relatively new. It was initially observed and defined in the 1960s by Dr. Christian de Duve, who was awarded the Nobel Prize in Physiology or Medicine in 1974 (Nobel Media AB, 2019). De Duve was studying the distribution of enzymes around areas of cell fragmentation when he discovered certain enzymes were attacking protoplasmic components surrounding cells. To protect the cell from damage during the attack, they were confined within a membrane, similar to a bubble. He named these bubbles lysosomes and characterized them like a cell's digestive system.

With his more significant understanding of lysosomes, he was able to go on to name the process of autophagy. Autophagy, he says, is:

Self-eating by cells. It's a mechanism whereby small bits of the cell are segregated - it's a complex mechanism - separated within a membrane and then conveyed to lysosomes for breakdown. So this is autophagy - self-eating - is one of the tools whereby cells degrade their substance and replace it. So it's part of turnover (Web of Stories - Life Stories of Remarkable People, 2017).

Along with Albert Claude and George E Palade, the two other men he shared the Nobel Prize with, de Duve is credited as being highly influential in the creation of the new field of cell biology.

Many years later, Yoshinori Ohsumi followed in his footsteps, winning the Nobel Prize in Physiology or Medicine in 2016 for "his discoveries of mechanisms for autophagy" (Nobel Media AB, 2019).

Dr. Ohsumi volunteered to spearhead research in the very uncompetitive field of vacuoles in yeast. Most scientists at the time were uninterested in exploring what was commonly thought to be the garbage dumps of cells.

He believed then what is widely agreed upon now: The degradation process in our bodies is just as necessary as the process of synthesis.

Thanks to his research, we understand that every process in our bodies relies on autophagy for survival, showing us how cells react to and handle malnourishment, infections, and certain diseases.

Cellular Recycling 101

Everything about being alive causes damage to our cells, even processes that are essential to our survival.

Try imagining every one of your cells as minuscule humans, each with unique and specialized jobs to do. They go to work each day and work very hard to keep you alive.

Just as physical, manual labor will cause some amount of damage to your body, the work that cells do causes typical damage to them throughout their lifespan.

Add to that any damage you inflict upon your body. Breathing in polluted air, ingesting toxins, and injuring yourself affects specific individual cells in your body. Bacteria and viruses also contribute to the daily damage that cells suffer.

Cells have a hard life. To survive and keep your entire body alive, they must have a way to heal themselves.

We've already discussed mitosis, the process by which cells duplicate themselves and divide to help you grow and heal.

But some cells don't have that ability.

Humans would have very short lifespans if the brain and heart cells didn't have another way to heal themselves from damage.

Autophagy provides a backup or alternative to cell division: cellular recycling.

To understand how and why cellular recycling is crucial to our survival, we first have to know how the cells in our bodies get the power required to do their jobs.

Your Digestive System

Your digestive system uses a variety of acids and enzymes to take what you eat and disassemble it so that it can be absorbed and used by our bodies.

All food is made up of 3 essential macronutrients: carbohydrates, proteins, and fats.

For anyone following the Standard American Diet (SAD), the majority of your food is carbs, which breaks down into glucose quickly, using enzymes in your saliva. Glucose then, is the primary source of energy that your body uses to power its cells.

The next part of the digestive process that we're interested in occurs in your stomach. The digestive acids and enzymes in your stomach first dissolve any large chunks of food and kill any bacteria that shouldn't be there. Then an enzyme called pepsin breaks down the proteins in your food into even smaller components called amino acids.

Finally, fats are the last to be broken down, and this happens as what remains of your food leaves your stomach and enters your small intestine. Using bile that's waiting in your gallbladder, the fats that you've ingested get emulsified and reduced to fatty acids and monoglycerides, which can finally be absorbed and used to power your cells.

Of course, there is a lot more to digestion, but

concerning autophagy, this is all you need to know. To summarize, your digestive system will separate everything you eat into one of three macronutrients and then, at different phases, dissolves each of those macros into components that your cells can absorb and use for power.

Carbohydrates digest the quickest, making glucose the first energy supply your body will pull from. Next to be rendered are proteins, providing amino acids to your cells. And finally, taking the longest to break down are fats, which are composed of fatty acids.

All of these nutrients are required to make sure your body not only has a constant source of energy to keep you alive, but they also provide you with everything you need to stay healthy and efficient.

When all that is left of the food you ate is glucose, amino acids, and fatty acids, your metabolic system gets to work, turning these components into energy for your cells.

Your Metabolic System

Most people know that the human body is primarily made up of water.

The next contributor is protein, making up about 17% of the total mass of a healthy person.

Part of this protein makes up your muscles, of course, but a great deal of it is housed in your neurons, blood, and every single one of your cells.

Fats also make up about 16% of your body; if you're at a healthy weight, this number fluctuates a great deal and is usually higher in women.

There are also minerals like calcium and iron, which make up about 4% of your total mass.

Only about 1% of your body, however, is made up of carbohydrates.

Isn't it fascinating that the macronutrient that we eat the most of actually account for the least amount of our mass, by a significant margin?

The reason for this is simple: it's consumed and used for energy faster, whereas proteins and fats get stored for use in the future, when and if the body's supply of carbs gets cut off.

Your metabolic system is responsible for every biochemical reaction that happens inside your body, but most importantly is the force behind the anabolic and catabolic reactions.

Anabolism consumes the energy your digestive system prepared and uses it to rebuild the proteins, fats, and carbs that make up your cells.

Catabolism is the release of this energy from your cells as they do their jobs and make sure your body functions as it should.

Cellular Respiration & Protein Synthesis

Each of the three macronutrients has its primary functions within your body.

The majority of what we eat becomes glucose. Cellular respiration adds oxygen to the glucose molecule and converts it to carbon dioxide, water, and energy.

Each of our cells has organelles inside of them called mitochondria. These organelles are responsible for taking that energy and storing it as adenosine triphosphate (ATP). ATP is the final product that your cells use to drive anabolic reactions.

ATP cannot be stored as ATP, however, so if you end up with leftovers, it gets converted into fat or glycogen.

Proteins mainly do everything else. Remember,

our body is approximately 17% protein, and thanks to a regular cycle of cell death, almost all of that protein is replaced every 2 – 3 months.

We need to produce a substantial amount of protein to meet these demands.

Our bodies require 200 – 300 grams of protein each day to continue using our muscles so we can move around as we need to, but also to build new cells to replace old and damaged ones.

According to the CDC (2017), in the USA, adults are getting between 15.6% - 16.1% of their daily calories from protein. In a diet of 2200 calories per day, this works out to about 350 calories or 88 grams of protein.

If we need up to 300 grams of protein each day to function, but we're taking in less than 90 on average, where is the rest coming from?

The Deep Science of Autophagy

Finally, we have come back to our primary topic: autophagy.

To make up the extra 100 – 200 grams of protein, your body will start to recycle other materials that are readily available and not currently being used.

Some level of cellular recycling is continuously occurring in your body at all times.

The official medical definition of autophagy is "digestion of cellular constituents by enzymes of the same cell" ("Autophagy," 2019).

In other words, autophagy is a metabolic process in which cells that are starved for energy use enzymes to break down their damaged components and convert the waste into nutrients that they can use instead, prolonging their life.

It's the cell's ultimate survival mechanism.

When a cell is starved for energy, it will look around itself to find anything unnecessary to its survival that it can use to degrade and recycle, including damaged or misfolded proteins and protein aggregates or certain bacteria and viruses.

Because food has become so available and plentiful, however, the natural rhythm of autophagy has become dysregulated in many people. It has become lazy, and it will clean up only as much internal debris as is necessary.

When you fast, which we'll get into in more detail in future chapters, you aren't even providing your body with the 80 - 90 grams or so that it is used to, yet the demand for new protein in your cells remains the same.

By placing more stress on your body, your autophagic processes kick into overdrive to keep the mandatory creation of new cells occurring. It is not only good news for keeping you alive, but it also keeps you healthier in the process, because more potentially damaging materials lingering in your body are recycled.

Some of the materials that your body will recycle include viruses, unwanted bacteria, remnants of dead or damaged cells, and even, potentially, cancer cells. Removing these threats to our health has numerous priceless benefits.

Compounding the benefits of removing and recycling dangerous debris inside our bodies is the fact that, once the garbage is gone, each cell and tissue in our body can work more efficiently simply because now their workspace is cleaner.

In order to begin the recycling process, your cell must separate the damaged components first. How this task is accomplished sets apart the three main levels or types of autophagy.

Macro, Micro, and Chaperone Mediated Autophagy

Macro-autophagy deals with large organisms that need to be broken down into smaller components to be converted to energy.

The cell first has to separate the unwanted materials from the healthy parts of the cell. Whatever is to be recycled gets pushed outside and encased in an autophagosome.

Imagine rounding up all the recyclable materials lying around your house and putting them outside your front door. Instead of being picked up by the recycling company, however, they get degraded immediately, right there on your doorstep.

In the first chapter, we discussed lysosomes, which were discovered by de Duve in the 60s, and began the field of research in autophagy.

Lysosomes are mostly little bubbles filled with enzymes. These enzymes can degrade nearly anything, including whatever it finds inside each autophagosome.

What the cell is now left with are the main building blocks of all organisms: proteins, fats, and carbs.

Within the process of macro-autophagy, there are two selection processes.

The cell can either go through a bulk process, where it recycles everything it can all at once or a selective process.

If it can be selective, it will choose only one type of material to recycle. When a fat cell is used, this is called lipophagy. The degradation of mitochondria is mitophagy, and when your body uses dead or infected microbes, it is called xenophagy (Dr.Education - FITNESS & NUTRITION, 2019).

Micro-autophagy applies to organisms that are small enough that they don't require an autophagosome but can be directly engulfed, digested, and converted into energy.

Chaperone-Mediated Autophagy (CMA) is the most selective form of this metabolic process, and it targets only particular amino acids and substrates and is also a direct process.

To avoid confusion and unnecessary complication of an already dense topic, for the rest of this book, we won't distinguish between the types of autophagy. When the autophagic process is triggered in any way, the appropriate process will take place.

Imagine cooking an elaborate dinner every night of the week, but never cleaning up afterward. Not only will you be creating a breeding ground for dangerous bacteria, but it's also going to become more inconvenient and difficult to get your cooking done as dishes pile up on your counters, and you have fewer tools to work with.

After a week of cooking, if you take the time to clean, the next time you cook, the process will be much more efficient.

Periodically stressing your body to the point where autophagy is induced will have a similar effect.

If, however, you clean your kitchen regularly, your cooking process will always be at maximum efficiency. Of course, accidents will still happen, and a clean kitchen is no guarantee that every meal will come out perfect, but it certainly does set you up for success.

Once your autophagic system is running optimally, you want to be sure to maintain the environment for the best results, which means not falling back into bad habits.

Later in the book, we'll discuss exactly how you can kickstart the process of autophagy as well as help you develop sustainable lifestyle changes to maintain healthy levels of autophagy operating at all times to maximize your probability of life-long health.

The Fountain of Youth

D.R Krauz

Chapter 2:

Dig In Before You Dive In

The more you understand about how your body works, the better equipped you'll be to support it.

Autophagy is a subject that some of the brightest minds on earth are still trying to understand, and it can be confusing and overwhelming. It can also be one of the most powerful resources you can harness to keep your body healthy and protected against chronic diseases proactively.

This chapter will discuss more about how autophagy relates to anti-aging, weight loss, and disease prevention. Of course, this will not be an exhaustive account of the subject, but it will arm you with enough information to help you apply specific principles to your own life.

More importantly, understanding why autophagy is so crucial to your health will help you stay true to any lifestyle changes you decide to adopt to maximize the benefits of this biological process.

What Does Autophagy Do, Really

One way to think of autophagy is to imagine an evolutionary, survival of the fittest battle happening in your body when resources get low.

Each one of the trillions of cells in your body needs energy to survive. They can get this energy either from the food you eat or from what is stored in your fat cells.

When both those supplies are tapped out, an enzyme called AMP-protein kinase (AMPK) is stimulated, which happens when you're in a caloric deficit due to either fasting or exercise.

Autophagy comes to the rescue, helping to ensure the survival of a starved but otherwise healthy cell by finding and using anything it can to convert to energy. Through this process, autophagy recycles unnecessary, and damaged products left over in the body, even protein aggregates or bacteria invading viruses.

Autophagy can even trigger a cell's death if that cell has finished its purpose and come to the end of its lifespan. The cell's parts will then be recycled and put to use in more efficient ways.

It's important to note that cells die in other ways, as well.

Apoptosis is a programmed cell death that might happen as a sort of self-destructive suicide if the cell knows it is dangerous to the body, or it might occur when the cell has simply fulfilled its purpose in life. Necrosis happens when your cell dies of unnatural causes such as infection or trauma.

You can also lose cells to dysregulated autophagy, when the process starts to break down healthy, functioning cells, leaving the organ that it belongs to vulnerable to disease. As you might expect, we want to prevent our autophagic system from becoming dysregulated, and we do that by triggering it more often. Autophagy breaks down as we age, so if we can protect our cells from aging prematurely, we'll preserve our healthy autophagic response.

Where Does The Damage Come From

You might be wondering why you have all these damaged and dangerous cell pieces in your body in the first place.

Damage happens from the simple fact of living

and is compounded by any stress that we experience.

For instance, our metabolism, the system that converts food to energy and keeps us alive, causes damage in our body both by working so hard to get the job done, as well as by leaving by-products and tiny bits of leftovers laying around.

An average, healthy level of stress is actually beneficial and helps us become stronger and more resistant to stress in the future.

Muscles grow by sustaining specific amounts of damage that is then repaired, leaving it bigger and stronger than before.

Abnormal stress causes more significant damage. Things like environmental toxins and chemicals, chronic stress, a poor diet, and chronic poor-quality sleep all create damage inside our bodies that builds up if it isn't effectively cleaned out. This buildup will continue to compound as we age, leading to a host of diseases.

Autophagy is the natural process that takes dead and damaged cells, recycles the leftovers, and renews and reinforces healthy cells that need repair and stimulates the production of new healthy cells.

It's triggered when there isn't enough energy in the form of food, coming into the body to sustain healthy function. Old, weak, and damaged cells can convert into energy in times of need.

Autophagy is also thought to have a healing trigger when the body is attacked by disease, infection, or injury. Depending on the level of the threat, the body will temporarily disrupt normal function to non-essential processes like digestion and cognition to target as much energy as possible to the specific cells that need healing.

Sick cells can then use autophagy to survive, removing the dangerous intracellular growth, bacteria, or virus.

The Implications of Autophagy

Now that you know how autophagy works inside your body, it's time to understand what the implications of this process are.

Autophagy has many known and suspected benefits. The fields of research that are particularly interested in its activity include aging, detoxification, immunity, and brain health. Together, these categories cover most, if not all, health issues that plague humans across the world.

Dr. William Dunn has been studying autophagy for over 30 years, with the express goal of learning how to turn autophagy on and off. With this ability, he believes we can find a cure for cancer, ensure life-long heart health, and even activate anti-aging properties (Whittel, 2019).

Disease Prevention

For most diseases, the path to recovery through autophagy is to use the metabolic process to clear away toxins, chemicals, bacteria, and other organisms before they can become harmful to our bodies.

In organs where cells do not divide, such as our heart, for example, autophagy is even more critical. Our hearts work very hard, with no little rest, throughout our entire lives. This regular, healthy stress still causes damage to our cells.

The cells in our hearts do not divide, which means they cannot repair themselves if or when they're damaged. They also use a great deal of ATP to keep themselves running around the clock, which ends up making the mitochondria in your heart cells age faster than in most other cells of your body.

When autophagy is operating as designed to, the damaged organelles in your heart cells will be cleared out regularly. If they aren't, they'll accumulate and build-up, leading to disease. If autophagy is dysregulated, you'll be at a higher risk for heart disease.

Similarly, most chronic and degenerative diseases are the result of chronic inflammation, which is triggered, in part, when we have too many toxins, irritants, and damaged cells in our body. When autophagy is operating to its highest potential, inflammation should come and go, but only when necessary, reducing the risk of nearly all diseases substantially.

The research hasn't found any guarantees yet, but autophagy is a subject with incredible potential to treat, cure, and prevent many major diseases.

A Cure for Cancer

Autophagy's relationship to cancer has drawn the attention of countless studies because, in this area, it seems to be a double-edged sword.

In the 1930s, yet another Nobel Prize winner, Otto Heinrich Warburg's research on respiratory enzymes, set the foundations for what we now understand about cellular metabolism and respiration. He was able to prove that cancer cells can survive and even grow when they're deprived of oxygen (Nobel Media AB, 2019).

He also discovered that cancer cells have unique feeding preferences. Healthy cells need your mitochondria to go through a 4-stage process that converts glucose to ATP. Cancer cells prefer glucose to ferment, rather than oxidize. For this reason, cancer cells tend to be seen growing in areas where mitochondria are damaged, and there is some evidence that cancer cells are even able to cause this dysfunction to boost their development. This phenomenon is known as the Warburg Effect.

Thomas Seyfried, a biochemical geneticist, has been studying this for more than 30 years. He developed what is called the Glucose Ketone Index (GKI) and found that when he was able to establish a balanced ratio of glucose and ketones in the blood of humans and mice with brain tumors, he saw a reduction in the growth of tumors. As glucose increased, the tumors would begin growing again (Meidenbauer et al., 2015).

To give you an idea, someone who is following a Standard American Diet will typically have a GKI ratio in the range of 30 to 50, which provides plenty of glucose for the development of cancer cells. As a person fasts or converts to a ketogenic diet, the ratio will balance itself out, coming closer to the desired 1:1 ratio. According to Seyfried, this is the therapeutic zone for reversing cancer, and it is also a reliable indicator for measuring autophagy.

In various other studies, cancer cells have been observed using the power of autophagy to feed themselves and grow more quickly. Cancerous tumors tend to grow dangerously fast, mainly because they're masters at confiscating the energy nearby to feed themselves. It's possible that, if a cancer cell has starved its immediate area of energy, it will stimulate and use the power of autophagy to break down material nearby, creating a new source of energy for itself.

Other studies have observed cancer cells shutting off the process of autophagy to protect themselves from being attacked.

And finally, some research is hopeful that autophagy will be able to recognize and target cancer cells before they ever have a chance to multiply and become a threat (Galluzzi et al., 2015).

Continued research in autophagy's role in cancer development and treatment is fascinating and controversial.

Nevertheless, there are other important areas of health where autophagy has already proven to have results.

Anti-Aging, Healthy Weight Loss & Brain Protection

When we talked about cellular respiration earlier, you were introduced to mitochondria, the organelles in your cells that convert glucose to ATP. It is responsible for about 95% of energy creation.

Mitochondria tend to be very sensitive and age more quickly than the other parts of your cells, causing breakdowns that are recognized as signs of aging.

Autophagy can repair mitochondria, helping them live longer, and contributing to the anti-aging properties it is so well known.

Autophagy assists healthy weight loss as well. First and foremost, it clears your body of waste. Broken and damaged cells take up unnecessary space inside your body, contributing to mass, however minuscule. Toxins that your body can't metabolize are often stored in fat cells, also contributing to weight gain. And unhealthy bacteria, viruses, and damaged material that lead to diseases cause inflammation and unwanted growths in your body. Get rid of all that through the process of autophagy, and you will also be removing unnecessary weight.

On a much grander scale, however, autophagy assists with healthy weight loss by turning your body into a fat-burning machine. You've probably heard similar promises about certain kinds of exercise or the ketogenic diet, both of which we're going to discuss in-depth in later chapters. For now, suffice it to say, the rumors are true, and if you can burn more fat, you will lose weight faster. If you effectively condition your body to continue burning fat, you will keep the weight off long-term, as opposed to most dieting results.

In terms of protecting your brain, a properly functioning autophagic response is not only incredibly beneficial but also necessary.

Your brain is unique compared to the rest of your body.

Your muscles are designed to be damaged and

repaired. Inflammation and lactic acid work together to restore the micro-tears caused by exercise and regular use, and this repair job makes your muscles stronger.

Your brain does not work the same way.

It doesn't have a built-in repair system and, just as your heart cells do not divide, neither do your brain cells. Instead, your brain is protected very well by your skull, explicitly designed to keep your brain from ever sustaining damage.

Of course, as we know, accidents happen.

Without a repair process in place and lacking the ability to duplicate cells to replace damaged ones, autophagy becomes even more critical to the health of your brain.

Autophagy is essential to clean up dead cells, toxins, and other debris that accumulates in your brain. Short term fasting is one of the most effective ways to induce autophagy in your brain (Alirezaei et al., 2010).

We'll talk more about ketones later in the book. Still, for now, it's also important to know that when we induce autophagy, ketones replace glucose as the primary source of nutrition for your brain, which reduces inflammation.

This technique is an effective strategy for healing from traumatic brain injuries, as well as protecting against degenerative diseases such as Alzheimer's and Parkinson's, which are caused by the accumulation of plaque on your brain cells.

Autophagy working in your brain can also have the simple benefit of helping you stay focused and sharp.

D.R Krauz

Chapter 3:

Truth or Dire?

Any new parent knows just how important growth is. How quickly a baby grows is tracked almost obsessively as a measure of health.

For the young, growth is seen as a sign of health and development, especially when the growth remains proportionate. The rate at which a child grows taller should be roughly proportionate to the rate at which they put on weight and muscle, and their bones and organs need to grow proportionately to support their new height and weight. It's a delicate balance, but in a healthy child, the balance is maintained naturally.

Once we reach adulthood, however, growth stops being a sign of health. At a certain point in every person's life, we stop growing taller. If we continue to grow, it will inherently be disproportionate and out of balance.

Growth, as an adult, is a precursor to or sign of

disease.

Obesity is the most apparent form of excessive growth, but cancerous tumors and enlarged organs are also extremely dangerous forms of growth.

Many diseases are caused by a build-up of plaque, including cardiovascular disease and neurological disorders.

Autophagy is one of the ways a healthy body maintains balance and protects you against excessive growth.

Losing Weight with Autophagy

Before we dive in, it's essential to make sure you not only understand but believe in one specific fact about weight management: weight and health are not mutually exclusive. Weight is not a guaranteed indicator of health or disease.

There are plenty of people in the world who are technically at their ideal body weight but are in worse health than others who are technically considered overweight.

Weight is one indicator of health, but it is not the only factor you have to consider. When you have the goal of losing weight, you should approach the process with your overall health in mind, also, with a good understanding of how your body was designed to operate.

That being said, if you've been struggling to manage your weight over the years, adapting your diet and exercise habits to induce autophagy is a very effective way to lose the extra weight and keep it off.

A lot of the weight management benefits of autophagy happen in the liver. If your body is maintaining a high level of autophagy, your clean and healthy liver will upregulate something called lipolysis, which is a fancy way of saying fat burning.

Regardless of how you stimulate autophagy, the results lead to more effective fat burning, which, as you can imagine, is helpful for weight loss.

Calories In Vs. Calories Out

For years we've been told that the secret to weight management is to make sure that the number of calories you put into your body is equal to or less than the number of calories you use daily.

It is not the whole story.

First of all, highly processed foods soaked in chemicals, hormones, pesticides, and more toxins are given a calorie count that only considers macronutrients. It does not account for the fact that all those chemicals, hormones, and other toxins will likely remain inside your body, encased in fat cells, because your body doesn't know what to do with them.

Moreover, as we've already discussed, the types of calories we eat and the timing in which we eat them affects our insulin response. When we become insulin resistant, our body starts to store more fat. It has more to do with having too much glucose in our system than with having too many calories.

Changing what kind and quality of calories we consume will have as big of an impact and more lasting results than merely reducing the number of calories we consume.

Modern Lifestyles - Blessing or Curse

Living in the 21st century comes with a lot of perks, especially when compared to how hard life was 100 or 200 years ago.

Life today is all about convenience.

Technological advancements allow us to violate the laws of nature to feel more comfortable. Unfortunately, this comfort is killing us.

Human bodies were designed to eat, move, and sleep, and we can do each of those things very efficiently.

Historically we ate when food was available, though we were forced to work hard to get it. We were naturally going through stages of feasting and famine.

Humans moved to stay safe, escape from predators, build a shelter to protect us from exposure to the elements, and hunt and gather food.

Even our sleep used to be regulated by the natural rise and fall of the sun.

Modern advancements have ensured that food is plentiful and easy to prepare. Machines and electronics allow us the luxury of being mainly sedentary, and we can even sleep whenever we feel like it or have time for it, thanks to electric lights.

These modern advancements have changed how we live, but they haven't altered how we were designed to live.

There are many, many benefits to living in the modern world, not least of which is decreasing starvation rates and cures to many diseases that used to be life-threatening.

Instead, we have rising rates of deaths and diseases caused, in large part, by over-consumption of convenient, junk food.

In essence, our built-in, naturally occurring system of preventative health has been superseded by our modern system of fixing things only when they break, pitting medications and surgeries against disease.

On the flip side, modern discoveries in scientific fields like autophagy are leading the way to discover how to reverse these downfalls while still enjoying all the perks.

Truths and Myths of Autophagy

Since Ohsumi's discoveries, autophagy has become a hot topic in the scientific and medical communities. Whenever something new is discovered that has the impressive potential that autophagy has, it takes on mythical proportions.

And with that comes a great deal of misunderstanding and mistruth. Before we explain how you can harness the power of autophagy, it is prudent to understand what is and is not expected or achievable.

Timed Starvation

Many so-called experts will tell you that a single 24-hour fast will help you live forever, and others who are adamant that you need to starve yourself for 3 - 5 days, sometimes even longer, to trigger autophagy.

Neither of those myths is strictly correct.

First, it's helpful to dispel the idea that autophagy is synonymous with starvation. Not consuming energy is not the same thing as starving. Your body always has stored reserves of energy to pull from, and therefore won't truly start starving until those reserves are entirely depleted.

As we've already discussed, your digestive system can take anywhere from 4 - 8 hours to completely break down and process your food. It means that from the time you eat your last meal, you may feel like you're fasting, but your body still has up to 8 hours worth of energy to consume. That leaves only 16 hours of nutrition deprived stress for your body to withstand within a 24 hour fast.

There is plenty of proven benefits to fasting for 24 hours or even fasting for shorter periods through different varieties of intermittent fasting.

Autophagy may be triggered within that 24-hour window, but it is unreasonable to assume everyone will see noticeable effects in such a short period.

At the other end of the spectrum, you don't necessarily need to avoid eating for days at a time to benefit from autophagic processes.

We'll talk more about this in the next chapter, but in order to turn on autophagy, your cells need to be energy deprived. Most carbohydrates turn into glucose after digestion, and glucose suppresses AMPK, which is pro-autophagy, and blood sugar levels rise.

Insulin is then released to balance your blood glucose, which in turn raises mTOR levels, inhibiting autophagy. It is a reasonably complex process, but for our purposes here, it's enough to know that autophagy will not be induced until the glucose in your body has been used up.

If you follow a diet that's low in carbs, you'll naturally have less glucose to convert to energy, and autophagy can be more easily stimulated. The

Standard American Diet (SAD) that a large portion of the world follows is high in carbohydrates, and from this position, it may take several days of fasting to trigger autophagy.

However, a moderate protein and high-fat diet will allow you to induce autophagy much more quickly.

Perfect Weight Loss

One of the reasons autophagy has picked up a lot of press in the past few years is because people who are following a plan to induce and benefit from autophagy see consistent and sustainable weight management results.

A healthy body will naturally regulate its own weight.

As we discussed earlier, too much growth as a full-grown adult leads to disease, so it follows that if your body's natural process of recycling is healthy, you will not have excessive growth, including holding onto too much weight.

Autophagy is not, however, a miracle cure or a diet you can follow for overnight success.

If your weight is already an issue, just like with

any other healthy plan to lose weight, it will take time.

If you're currently at a healthy weight, making lifestyle changes to support your autophagic process will help you stay that way.

Another myth that has been circulated is that if you lose a great deal of weight following an eating and exercise plan designed to induce autophagy, the recycling process will protect you from sagging skin and wrinkles, a common byproduct of extreme weight loss.

While it is true that autophagy helps keep your skin healthy, elastic, and youthful, there are limits to what you should expect.

When you retain extra weight for a long time, your body creates more skin cells to compensate. Some of those cells will be stretched or otherwise damaged and may be targeted by autophagy for clean up, but many of them will be healthy cells.

As you lose weight, you'll end up with a surplus of healthy skin cells. Depending on how much weight you lose, they may not have anywhere to go, so they'll end up sagging.

Over time, the surplus cells won't be replaced as they die, and gradually the sagging skin will reduce, especially if you continue to support healthy autophagy. Your new skin cells retain their elasticity well.

But the timing will not necessarily line up with your weight loss and autophagy cannot guarantee you complete protection from sagging skin and wrinkles.

Additional Myths

Some believe that fasting is the only way to induce autophagy, and others imagine that any amount of calorie restriction will ignite autophagy. Some experts suggest that maintaining a low-carb diet indefinitely will ensure autophagy also operates forever.

Some claim that autophagy can cure all diseases and reverse aging. Others will tell you that it's completely unproven and dangerous, potentially even cancer-inducing.

The truth is autophagy will work best in a healthy body, and it will work hard to keep your body healthy. It is one very complicated biological system out of the many that keep us alive and functioning.

Autophagy shouldn't be approached like a miracle

cure; nevertheless, we can't ignore its benefits either.

Autophagy will help with immunity, anti-aging, anti-inflammation, longevity, healing, and recycling.

We still have a lot to learn about it, but what we do know is that if you make some strategic lifestyle changes to support your natural autophagic processes, you will be stacking the deck in your favor.

The Fountain of Youth

D.R Krauz

Chapter 4:

So You Think You Can Fast?

Since Ohsumi's Nobel Prize, many researchers, scientists, and doctors have begun to focus their research on autophagy. If we can learn how to turn this process on and off at will and target it to specific organs or cells, there's a good chance that many diseases can be cured or, at the very least, treated more effectively.

To date, most experts agree that there are three very effective ways to trigger your body's normal autophagy process: exercise, ketosis, and fasting.

In an interview on the subject, Christiaan Leeuwenburgh, Ph.D., shares his process to induce the anti-aging properties of autophagy on a daily basis (Whittel, 2019). He practices intermittent fasting regularly, so he doesn't eat upon first waking up. Instead, he incorporates movement and exercise into his morning routine, to stress his muscles and stimulate the need for additional energy production.

Leeuwenburgh stresses the importance of staying hydrated, especially while in a fasted state. His overall goal is to stimulate his metabolism strategically to trigger the body's natural defenses - namely, autophagy.

Let's take a closer look at exactly why exercise, ketosis, and fasting are the best ways to kickstart autophagy in your own body.

Exercise

As we've discussed previously, autophagy responds when your body is under stress and needs a fresh burst of energy to cope.

To exercise is a form of healthy stress that produces an autophagic response.

Research shows that when your muscles are not only rapidly burning energy but also sustaining micro-injuries, autophagy is induced. But it isn't just called to repair the muscle. Once it starts, it continues to work in multiple systems of your body, including skeletal and cardiac muscles in mice test subjects (He et al., 2012), but also in other areas, such as your liver cells (Chun et al., 2017).

Participating in a moderate level of exercise on a consistent basis is well known to have a wide variety of health benefits. Now that we know it will also help stimulate the process of autophagy, there's even more reason to move your body wisely.

What Kind of Exercise Is Ideal

As long as you're moving your body, you're getting the benefits of exercise, right?

Wrong. There are plenty of ways you can ultimately do damage to your body by trying to do something healthy. There are even more ways you can work your body to exhaustion and see little to no beneficial results.

Most people exercise to lose weight or gain muscle, but both of those reasons are usually vanity goals more than they are health goals. When you think about exercising or working out, try to approach it from a health perspective instead.

Let's take a quick look at how people gain unhealthy amounts of weight in the first place.

Conventional wisdom suggests that weight gain occurs when you eat too much and exercise too little. Once you've gained weight, and especially if you're obese, you become insulin resistant and start suffering from metabolic diseases like Type 2 Diabetes and heart disease.

New research is flipping the equation.

Peter Attia has focused the majority of his medical career on studying the science of longevity. He suggests that when a body becomes insulin resistant, the cells start to ignore, or perhaps misunderstand, insulin's suggestion to burn energy and decide to store it as fat instead.

If you look at it this way, weight gain and obesity is a response or symptom of insulin resistance, not the other way around.

This makes the problem of insulin resistance much larger because currently, as a society, we blame the disease on the weight. But there are 30 million obese Americans without insulin resistance and 6 million lean Americans who do have insulin resistance. The first group doesn't appear to be at high-risk, whereas the lean people seem to be at an even greater risk for metabolic disease. Attia suggests this might be because their systems haven't figured out what to do with the energy when the cells stop responding to insulin (Ted, 2013).

With this in mind, exercising to lose weight isn't necessarily guaranteed to make you any healthier.

There is a difference between eating too much food and having too much glucose in your blood, so overeating and not exercising enough may not be the problem. Eating too many carbohydrates that convert quickly to glucose might be the culprit.

But what does all this have to do with autophagy and exercise?

Well, in part, it should affect how you think about why you're exercising. If you stop focusing on losing weight and start focusing on balancing your blood sugar, the type of exercise you practice might change.

Aerobic exercise, or steady and consistent cardio, increases your need for oxygen, using it to sustain your level of activity without needing another energy source.

When you participate in anaerobic exercise, oxygen isn't enough, and it starts to burn glucose as well, which creates the by-product lactic acid. If you start to feel your muscles burn, that's the lactic acid talking.

High-Intensity Interval Training (HIIT) benefits

both aerobic and anaerobic functioning and has been shown to get better results in both areas in a shorter period of time. HIIT is a style of training where you push yourself to 80+% of your maximum heart rate for a short period, and follow it with a recovery interval of around 40% of your maximum heart rate for an even shorter period, and then you repeat the process.

A common example is a 30-second sprint followed by a 10-second recovery, repeated three times. You would then get a rest period of 2 minutes, and then move on to a new set of intervals.

So which type of exercise is best?

Put, HIIT allows you to get all the benefits of a complete aerobic and anaerobic workout plan in a shorter period of time. For this reason, it will help you get into the autophagic zone without pushing you too far and causing more damage. Less time working out with better overall results is ideal, wouldn't you agree?

Most experts do, but let's see why.

How Does Exercise Induce Autophagy

We've talked about inducing autophagy through

stress on your body and calorie restriction; both play a part in how exercise triggers the process.

But we've also mentioned that autophagy is a process that occurs regularly, and becomes dangerous if it gets dysregulated, or doesn't function properly.

What we haven't yet talked about is how autophagy is inhibited.

We know that the enzyme AMPK is stimulated when you experience caloric restriction, and the more AMPK there is present, the more autophagy will happen. It is the anabolic reaction.

As you know, for every anabolic reaction, there is going to be a catabolic one. When you're in a state of excess calories, a protein called Mammalian Target of Rapamycin (mTOR) is turned on, which inhibits the formation of autophagosomes, making autophagy impossible.

Aerobic exercise stimulates AMPK, whereas resistance training stimulates mTOR, which is associated with growth hormones. However, without autophagy, you can't build muscle either, because the damage would never be fully repaired and inflammation would be too disruptive, so even though mTOR is present, autophagy is as well.

Excessive strength-training can throw autophagy into overdrive on the other side of the spectrum, causing muscle atrophy.

Resistance training, in conjunction with fasting, can provide the right balance of autophagy to mTOR production, but so can HIIT.

Again, High-Intensity Interval Training gives you all the benefits of both aerobic and anaerobic exercise - and potentially even more - in less time. It means you're less likely to overtrain and cause more damage (Land, 2019).

Additional Benefits to Exercising

Even if we agree that weight isn't the most important reason for you to exercise, there are plenty of additional benefits to moving your body.

Interestingly, many of the benefits associated with exercise are similar to the benefits of autophagy itself.

Exercise is a great way to combat disease, and it's been shown to reduce the risk of neurodegeneration, improve immune function, lower blood pressure, and even aid in cancer prevention.

It's also one of the best ways to stabilize your hormones, which, as we know, is part of the autophagic process. Still, it can also improve mood disorders like depression, anxiety, and even bipolar disorder.

Exercise, especially HIIT, releases Human Growth Hormone (HGH), which helps regulate body fat, develop lean muscle, and even improve bone density. HGH naturally declines as we age, so by producing more of it, you can reduce many effects of aging, such as osteoporosis and thin, papery, wrinkled skin.

In each of our cells, we normally have 23 pairs of chromosomes that carry our DNA. Each one of these chromosomes has a little cap on the end of it, called a telomere, protecting it from damage and degeneration. However, every time a cell duplicates itself, these telomeres get a tiny bit shorter. The older we get, the shorter our telomeres are, and the less protected our chromosomes become. High-intensity exercise has been shown to preserve telomere length, helping us slow the effects of getting older (Brigham Young University, 2017).

The more science applies itself to the question of

exercise, the more it appears that incorporating High-Intensity Interval Training (HIIT) is a great idea for many aspects of our health.

Fasting

We already know that autophagy is called to duty when your cells don't have access to enough energy to keep them working efficiently. Energy comes from the food we eat. If we're constantly eating, our cells will always have enough energy.

It sounds good in theory, but there are two main problems.

First, if autophagy is dysregulated, or isn't called to action often enough, the damaged, dead and unwanted material that gets leftover from normal metabolic processes and daily stress will never be removed. It will simply accumulate and eventually cause one kind of disease or breakdown or another.

The problem is compounded by the fact that our modern diet and lifestyles add to the number of toxins and chemicals polluting our bodies. Without autophagy, not only are we not removing the normal damage and waste from our cells, but we're also allowing the extra dose of damaging material to continue to wreak havoc inside of us.

The second main problem is that the pleasure of eating has turned us from a species that eats in order to live, to a species that lives to eat.

According to the World Health Organization, a fast-growing minority of earth's population is consuming more energy than they need, to a considerable degree. In 2016, 39% of adults were considered overweight, and of those adults, 13% were obese (World Health Organization 2016).

Monitoring the amount of energy we provide our cells is crucial to our health. As it turns out, regulating how often we provide energy to our cells can also make a significant impact on our health.

What Is Fasting

Fasting is simply not eating for some time. As an English speaker, you're no doubt familiar with the concept of breakfast. It was named as such because it's the meal in which you break your fast, or the time you were not eating, mainly because you were sleeping.

Most people will naturally fast for at least 8 hours a day.

Water fasting is one form of fasting in which you don't consume any calories for a set period, but you do drink water. Dry fasting means you don't drink any water either.

Between those two types of fasting, if your primary goal is to trigger autophagy, research shows that dry fasting is technically the better option.

Dry fasting burns fat cells more quickly because the body is forced to essentially squeeze water out of your fat cells to stay alive. The water it produces is very high quality, purified water, which is preferential for any healing that might be going on in your body.

Because you're burning through fat cells more quickly, the autophagy process will set in more quickly as well.

The counter-argument, however, is that you can't sustain dry fasting as long as you can a water fast. Dry fasting may work well on an intermittent schedule, but unless you're medically supervised and have significant experience with fasting, anything longer than 24 hours should be a water fast.

Any amount of time spent without food is

considered a fast, but keep in mind that your digestive system takes 4 - 6 hours to process any food you give it. So if you follow the average breakfast, lunch, snack, dinner meal plan, you will be feeding your body quicker than it can digest. If you add more snacks to the equation, you are setting yourself up for glucose storage.

For example, if you have breakfast at 8 am, you won't burn through that glucose until noon when you eat lunch. If you save dinner until 6 pm, there's a good chance you'll have run through your readily accessible energy, but barely. You haven't given your system a chance to do anything but digest and decide what to store as fat.

Then, your body is going to need the entire night to recover from the stress of the day. The more time you can fast after eating your final meal of the day, and before eating your first meal of the next day, the more time your body will have to focus its energy on tasks other than digestion.

How Does It Trigger Autophagy

The process of digestion is one of the most demanding on your body. As mentioned, our body has the best opportunity to do its repair work while we sleep, since we're not bombarding it with multiple other jobs to complete.

It should be a good enough incentive to get a solid 8 hours of restorative sleep every night.

Beyond the basics of digestion, caloric restriction is the most common and preferred way to kickstart the process of autophagy.

When you stop adding new sources of energy, insulin will drop and trigger growth hormones.

Your body's need to create new cells and repair tissue doesn't change just because you stop eating. A few non-essential systems may go on holiday, but for the most part, it's business as usual inside your body. The only difference is that without a new source of energy, your body has to get a lot better at cellular recycling.

You don't want to recycle protein, however, because that is what is used to create those new cells and repair that tissue, so the additional growth hormones protect your protein.

Autophagy is called in as backup.

It starts scouring your body for any debris or unnecessary molecule to recycle. Because of the enzymes in lysosomes, autophagy can break down nearly any substance in your body that shouldn't be there, including toxic material that was stored in fat because it didn't have anywhere else to go.

One of the downfalls of burning fat for fuel is that it can release all the foreign and potentially dangerous material that was hidden there for safekeeping. It may lead to detoxing as a negative side effect. When you go far enough into fasting and ketosis to trigger autophagy, it helps a great deal with these detoxing symptoms by recycling the toxins instead of letting them loose inside your body.

Remember that Nobel Prize winner Ohsumi discovered the mechanisms of autophagy because of his belief that the processes of degradation were just as important as the processes of synthesis. He was right, and the field of autophagy will be forever grateful for his diligence.

Additional Benefits to Fasting

One of the primary benefits of intermittent fasting is an improvement to your insulin response, which is a very significant factor in weight gain and most metabolic diseases like Type 2 diabetes. Every time you eat, your metabolism creates an insulin response.

Fasting also improves the health of your brain and your cognitive function.

Mark Mattson, professor of Neuroscience at Johns Hopkins University, studied the specific neurotrophic factors BDNF and FDF, which are proteins in the brain that help keep neurons strong and functioning well. He found that exercise and IF (Intermittent Fasting) helped increase these proteins and even stimulate the production of new nerve cells from stem cells (TEDex Talks, 2014).

Fasting causes oxidative stress, creating damage that needs to be repaired. In response, BDNF increases to repair the damage, making it even stronger for the trouble. This process is very similar to strengthening your muscles.

Fasting is also a great way to lose weight in a healthy, sustainable fashion, focusing on your nutrition at the same time. Reducing the amount of time you spend eating each day will naturally reduce the number of calories consumed. As mentioned at multiple other points in this book, calories are not all created equal, and you should be considering quality at least as carefully as you consider quantity.

If you are providing your body with less energy to

run on, it's crucial to make sure that the energy you do give it is very high quality. Stimulating autophagy is great, but it is only one way in which your body remains healthy.

Combining fasting with high-quality nutrition, full of vitamins and minerals, and low on chemicals and additives will help you feel great and look as good as you feel.

Once your body gets used to the new feeding schedule, and your insulin response is stabilized, you will notice that you don't feel the need to eat nearly as often as you did before. It helps make fasting a sustainable eating plan rather than a diet.

Diets are short term fixes with short term results. An eating plan is a lifestyle change with life-long effects.

Ketosis

As we already know, for most people, glucose is the first energy source that your body reaches for, and it's also the primary source of energy for your neurons and blood cells. Because glucose is so crucial to your survival, your body likes to maintain a very strategic blood glucose level of

70-100 mg/dL.

If you've eaten too many carbs, your blood glucose levels will rise. As your blood sugar rises, your pancreas is alerted, and it starts to release insulin.

Insulin moves glucose out of our blood and transfers it into storage, also known as fat cells.

As insulin removes the glucose from your blood and your cells continue to use what is left and available for energy, your blood sugar levels will drop.

Your pancreas is now called to release glucagon, which triggers your liver and adipose tissue to release their fat stores to send some of your stored glucose back into the blood.

It is the essential metabolic process that happens whenever you eat, especially when you eat a high carb diet such as the Standard American Diet (SAD).

Most of the cells in your body can either use glucose or ketones to convert to useable energy.

While your feeding patterns follow the Standard American Diet (SAD), your cells become accustomed to using carbs, but just because they're used to it, doesn't mean it's the only or best choice of fuel.

When you follow a low-carb, and high-fat diet, your body will get more practice burning fat for energy instead. It will use whatever resources it has to stay alive and well.

In 1921, endocrinologist Rollin Woodyatt made an extraordinary discovery. He discovered that three ketones (water-soluble compounds), acetone, beta-hydroxybutyrate, and acetoacetate, were produced by the liver when it was starved or if it only was fed by a diet rich in fat and low in carbs. Russel Wilder from the Mayo Clinic named this the Ketogenic Diet, also in 1921 (Mandal, 2019).

Gluconeogenesis is the process of breaking down non-carbohydrate sources, except for fatty acids, and ketogenesis breaks down fatty acids and amino acids. When both these processes occur, glucose is produced along with ketone bodies.

When your blood glucose levels and blood ketone levels dip below a 9 on the GKI, you will enter a state called ketosis.

How Does It Support Autophagy

Research has shown that autophagy is required

during the process of gluconeogenesis to maintain energy homeostasis, and therefore the process is triggered by the production of ketones (Takagi et al., 2016).

When it comes down to it, fasting will not trigger autophagy if you are not in a state of ketosis. If you are already fat-adapted, your body is used to being ketotic. It is probably close to ketosis already, the effects of autophagy will register much more quickly when combined with fasting.

As mentioned before, if your blood measures less than 9 on the GKI, you are considered in ketosis, which has an entire range of benefits on its own. We'll get into those in a moment.

You need to reach the therapeutic zone of ketosis in order to trigger autophagy, which occurs when your GKI balances out in the range of 1 -3.

If you fast while following a SAD, it could take 72 hours or more to reach this therapeutic range of ketosis. By following a low-carb diet regularly, you could reduce that period to 24 hours or less.

Being able to trigger autophagy quicker will give you many more opportunities to let it work on cleaning up your body, and it will be much easier to maintain in the long-term.

If you have to fast for five days every time you want to induce autophagy, it will be a significant ordeal each time. However, if you can start seeing benefits after 16 or 24 hours, the process will be much easier to repeat on occasion to reap the rewards.

Additional Benefits to Ketosis

The Ketogenic Diet originated in the 20s and 30s when it was used as a therapy for patients who have epilepsy. It was a convenient alternative to fasting, which had already been shown to be effective in treating those prone to epileptic seizures. It went out of fashion when anticonvulsant medications were developed; however, they were only effective in about 20-30% of people with epilepsy, so the diet was reintroduced as a management tool.

Continuing research has shown that more ketones are produced by medium-chain triglycerides (MCTs), a particular type of fat. Because they travel via the hepatic portal vein - a blood vessel that carries blood directly from the gastrointestinal tract, gallbladder, pancreas, and spleen to the liver - as opposed to the lymphatic system which caters to the entire body. The MCT Diet evolved from keto, in which dieters derive

60% of their calories from MCT oil.

Ketosis has also been shown to have incredibly useful results in managing diabetes.

People with diabetes either have trouble producing (Type 1) or responding to insulin (Type 2). The Keto diet has been shown to improve blood sugar control and reduce the requirements shouldered by insulin (Leow et al., 2018).

For Type 1 diabetics, ketosis could have significant side effects and should be approached quite carefully.

First, it's important to monitor carefully the amount of insulin taken because following a low-carb diet will reduce insulin requirements (Krebs et al., 2016). Studies have shown the Keto Diet to be effective in lowering blood sugar levels in people with both Type 1 and 2 diabetes. However, there is always the risk that without proper insulin management, blood sugar can fall too low and result in dizziness, confusion, and even loss of consciousness.

Next, it's important to understand the difference between Diabetic ketoacidosis (DKA) and Ketosis.

In a healthy person who eats a low-carb, high-fat diet, the body is shifted into nutritional ketosis and can start burning fat for energy.

Diabetic ketoacidosis, however, happens in a Type 1 diabetic when the lack of insulin forces a rapid rise in blood sugar and blood ketones, throwing off the pH in the blood and resulting in a life-threatening emergency.

In nutritional ketosis, only ketones are increased, not blood sugar, which doesn't disrupt the acid-base balance in your blood.

Being in ketosis has picked up a great deal of popularity for having fast and long-lasting weight loss results. Eliminating high-carb food options naturally reduces calories consumed, but increasing fat intake leaves dieters feeling satiated longer and reduces their overall appetite.

In general, it tends to be much easier to sustain long-term than severely calorie-restrictive diets.

There have been numerous other benefits associated with ketosis including, but not limited to: reduced risk of heart disease, more effective cancer treatment and slower tumor growth, protection against neurological degenerative disorders such as Alzheimer's and Parkinson's, as well as other neurological conditions such as epilepsy and brain damage, and improvements in hormonal conditions like PCOS and acne.

Is Long Term Ketosis Safe

The world seems to be split into two groups: those who swear by ketosis for life, and those who are convinced that eating so much fat must be terrible for your health.

The truth lies somewhere in the middle. As with most things, there are healthy fats and unhealthy fats, as well as limits to what is wise.

For many years there was a lot of fear-mongering around the subjects of fats and cholesterol, giving rise to an entire industry of fat-free and low-fat products. It was triggered by a rise in illnesses that began when people started to increase the amount of human-made fats they were eating, specifically margarine. It was made out to be a healthy, more convenient version of butter and shortening, which replaced the more natural lard.

Unfortunately, the type of fats people were eating wasn't considered. It was merely all labeled as evil.

People mistakenly believed that if you didn't eat fat, you couldn't get fat. Of course, over the years since, that theory has been proven false as obesity levels continued to rise.

The belief, however, is hard to shake. Even when people see results and feel great following a high-fat diet, they still have a hard time letting go of the fear.

Studies are now available that show that the amount of fat that is eaten has little relationship to weight or heart disease, but rather it's the type of fat that makes a difference. If you choose fats that are derived from whole foods and natural sources, you're eating as Mother Nature intended.

There is also an argument that your body prefers to convert carbs to glucose because it's easier. But just become something happens quicker in your body it does not necessarily make it a better process. If you begin eating a high-fat, low-carb diet, it will adjust, and as long as you are getting the right balance of nutrients and calories, there will be no problem converting enough fat into glucose to power all your cells.

If you eat natural, whole foods that fit within a Ketogenic diet, it can be not just safe, but healthy, to maintain long-term.

The Autophagy Lifestyle Planner

(<u>DO NOT</u> even consider inducing autophagy without proper planning...)

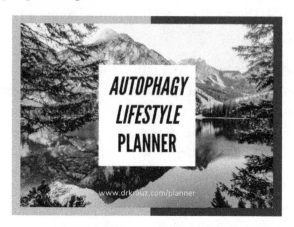

With the *Autophagy Lifestyle* Planner, you'll get:

➢ The **9 key elements** you cannot induce autophagy without.
➢ How to schedule them into your week, for maximum results.
➢ An effective way of keeping yourself accountable.

The last thing we want is for you to learn all the valuable insights contained in this book, but never be able to apply them.

To get your *Autophagy Lifestyle Planner,* visit the link: <u>www.drkrauz.com/planner</u>

The Fountain of Youth

D.R Krauz

Chapter 5:

If It Hurts, It Works (Or Not!)

In order to follow an autophagy inducing diet, it's just as important to focus on when, or how often, you eat as it is to pay attention to what you eat. It's possible to trigger the process of autophagy by fasting no matter what diet you're on. Still, the quickest route to autophagy comes when your body is already in a state of ketosis, which occurs when you follow a Ketogenic diet.

As you know, autophagy begins when cells in your body lose their constant source of easy energy, glucose. It moves into high gear when they've also eaten through the stores of glucose your body has on back up.

So getting autophagy started depends heavily on how much glucose you have on reserve. It doesn't just mean how much extra fat you have. It will also depend on how well your body does or does not respond to insulin.

Anyone following the Standard American Diet (SAD) is in a state of carbohydrate dependency, and many will have some level of insulin resistance. If you were to start fasting from this state, it could take up to 3 days for the main force of autophagy to be called to action.

However, if your body has had practice burning fat for fuel, known as being fat-adapted, which happens when you've been following a ketogenic diet for some time, your body will be primed for autophagy already. In this state, you could probably benefit from autophagy in as little as 16 to 24 hours of fasting.

Going from the SAD to a ketogenic diet overnight can be hard on your body and create a lot of unnecessary discomfort and digestive issues. It will help you to transition over time, cutting your carbs and increasing your intake of healthy fats progressively.

A low-carb diet brings the amount of energy you consume from carbs down to 20% of your overall calories, whereas a keto diet allows for only 5%. That is a drastic drop from an average of 50%, so it will take time to get to this stage, but the benefits are well worth it.

Once your body gets accustomed to the new diet,

you can work on the fasting as well, potentially working your way up with Intermittent Fasting (IF) and finally leading into longer fasts.

Now that you understand the general plan let's talk about specifics.

The Schedule: When to Eat

Even though this book comes out heavily in support of the benefits of fasting, you must approach this technique safely. It is not a good idea to go from a SAD where you're heavily dependent on carbohydrates and eating five or more times a day to immediately attempting a 7-day water fast.

That is very dangerous and not sustainable. Fasting is not a fast process.

If you take the time to help your body adapt to a new way of feeding, you will be able to enjoy long-term benefits in a safe and relatively comfortable manner.

If you are currently following a SAD – and it's called "standard" for a reason – your metabolic system has likely been conditioned to rely on regular feedings, sometimes upwards of 7 times a day.

Frequent, easy to digest meals were touted as the healthiest way to sustain energy for many years. Roughly the same number of years as the rate of obesity and metabolic diseases have been on the rise.

If you look at all the research shared in this book and through countless other sources, it becomes painfully obvious that this advice is flawed.

You've likely heard of sugar highs and crashes and understand how hard that is on your body. Carbohydrates, as you now know, are quickly converted to glucose, which is sugar. Even if you're not snacking on donuts and cookies, you're still putting your body on the same rollercoaster.

While it may sound counterintuitive at first, reducing the frequency of your eating patterns will help you stabilize your blood sugar levels and help you avoid the extreme highs and lows.

Intermittent Fasting (IF)

Intermittent Fasting (IF) is not a license to eat anything you want, no matter what you've heard online. Whenever something sounds too good to be true, it probably is.

Some foods are unhealthy and should not be part

of your eating plan. While eating nothing but junk food on an intermittent fasting schedule might be marginally better than eating nothing but junk food on an unregulated schedule, you're still going to be polluting your body with empty calories and harmful chemicals, additives, and toxins. Without a healthy supply of real, whole foods that are nutrient-dense, your body will disintegrate over time.

You need both macro and micronutrients to survive and thrive no matter how often you eat, so please don't consider intermittent fasting an unrestricted get out of jail free card.

There are many different ways to fast, but to save you from overwhelm, let's talk about the most popular options.

The most basic form of fasting is to stop eating for 24 hours. It can be done weekly, or monthly, or any time you decide, your internal systems could benefit from a spring clean. If you're used to feeding three or more times per day, it's a good idea to work your way up to a 24 hour fast using one or more of the other options.

The most popular form of Intermittent Fasting (IF) is time-restricted eating. In this option, you restrict your feeding window within a specified period per day, reducing the number of hours you allow yourself to consume calories as your body adapts. You can start on 12/12 and work your way up to 16/8, restricting your food intake to a window of only 8 hours each day, and fasting for the other 16 hours.

Many people find that following this pattern on a long-term basis helps keep them energized, since it naturally regulates blood sugar levels, and their caloric intake as well.

One Meal A Day (OMAD)

As you shrink your feeding window over time, you'll become more adapted to burning fat for fuel, and you may find yourself able to consume all of your calories for the day in one meal.

To make this a strategic health and weight management tool, you must work your way up to this stage gradually. If you try to do it all at once, your body will essentially go into shock, and try to conserve as much energy as possible, assuming the worst-case scenario.

If you teach your body to expect a single meal a day, it will have the confidence to continue using and processing your energy as usual.

Choosing to eat One Meal a Day (OMAD) is a relatively extreme form of intermittent fasting that, if done right, can be a very effective way to maximize the amount of healing your body has time to do.

It's one of the best ways to improve your insulin resistance and also reduces the amount of work your digestive and metabolic systems have to do. Instead of spending all day digesting and processing food, your body can focus on repairing the damage that has accumulated over the years.

Eating only once a day can be a way to restrict calories to induce autophagy, but it will also likely reduce the number of calories you consume, which will naturally lead to weight loss.

If you train your body to only expect food once per day, you'll eventually become accustomed to this, and hunger won't be an issue. However, the number of calories you can physically consume in a single meal is going to be limited, so naturally, you'll be inclined to take in fewer calories.

You must focus on the quality of your calories if you decide to try OMAD and make sure you still take in enough calories to keep your body functioning. Yes, this is a form of fasting, but you still want to be sure that overall, you aren't stressing your body too much.

Water Fasting – Rewards, Side Effects & Success Tips

Water fasting means that you survive on nothing but water for a set period. It could be 24 hours, or it could be 40 days.

Fasting has been practiced for religious and health reasons for as long as we have recorded history.

It's become trendy in recent times as a quick way to lose weight, and, though it might work, it's not a miracle cure and should only be practiced as part of an overall healthy lifestyle plan. A single water-fast might help you lose a few pounds, but as soon as you return to your old habits, the weight will come back and probably bring a few friends.

As part of a healthy lifestyle, however, a water fast can help you do more than lose weight.

We've talked about inducing autophagy, of course, as well as stabilizing blood sugar levels through fasting. The combination of these two results will help lower risks of metabolic diseases like diabetes and heart disease, among others.

One study demonstrated that water fasting could be an incredibly successful way to lower blood pressure, as well. One hundred seventy-four patients suffering from high blood pressure, at levels of 140/90 mm Hg and up, were able to reduce their blood pressure by an average of 37/13 mm Hg through a single, medically supervised 10-11 day water fast, with carefully regulated pre-fasting and refeeding periods (Goldhammer et al., 2001). Perhaps the most promising result of the study was that those who presented with the most severe hypertension saw the most significant reductions.

Notice that these results I just shared with you are from a medically supervised study. Long-term water fasting, anything over 72 hours, is not without its risks and should always be monitored for your safety.

Water fasting can be dangerous for pregnant women, children, and anyone with diabetes. If you have any history of disordered eating, long term fasting can trigger seriously harmful behaviors and should be avoided.

For healthy adults, however, water fasting beyond 24 hours may result in a few, relatively insignificant side effects, namely dizziness, weakness, and low energy. If you're planning a fast, it's a good idea to make sure you have the luxury of getting plenty of rest during this time. And don't forget to hydrate!

In order to get the most out of your fast, it's essential to plan your post-fasting feeding carefully. You shouldn't just return to regular eating habits immediately. Eating a big, heavy meal after a fast may be very hard on your digestive system and make you feel uncomfortable.

Instead, gradually introduce food back into your system. Try eating half an avocado, for example, and then waiting half an hour to an hour before continuing with your meal.

What breaks a fast? Anything that has calories.

A better answer to look for, however, is what you can actually eat or drink that won't compromise the benefits of the fast. To induce autophagy and improve insulin resistance, you can have water, black coffee, or tea.

You may also have items that won't trigger an insulin response. It might include minimal amounts of healthy fat, such as having a bulletproof coffee. Or you might want to put a little lemon or apple cider vinegar in your water. Fat has calories, so it will, technically, break your fast. But it really won't challenge the benefits of your fasting.

The Diet: What to Eat

Some of the most common mistakes people make when they attempt Intermittent Fasting (IF) or a Keto diet revolve around merely not understanding the macronutrients that they're eating. Too much or too little of any macronutrient is going to sabotage your efforts.

First, you want to make sure you're not eating too many carbs. Carbs and proteins, to a lesser degree, will trigger your insulin response and could end up storing the glucose instead of burning it as fuel.

It's also possible to eat too much fat or have too many calories. Just because you're reducing your feeding window through Intermittent Fasting (IF) doesn't mean you can completely ignore the volume of food that you're feeding your body.

On the flip side of that argument, you also want to make sure you don't eat too few calories. You always need to make sure your body has enough nutrition to stay healthy overall.

While you're fasting, it will help a great deal to make sure you're properly hydrated. It means drinking water as well as making sure you're getting enough electrolytes to maintain the fluid balance in your body. Salt has been given a bad reputation, but we need sodium to stay hydrated.

We already explained why it's important to choose whole, real foods over highly processed options to get the vital nutrition your body needs to operate effectively, regardless of when or how many calories you take in. Quality is the key to health.

The same will hold when it comes to following a ketogenic diet. A high-fat, moderate protein, low-carb diet is not a license to eat nothing but fried meat slathered in butter. You want to focus on high quality, nutrient-dense fats so that you can put your body into a state of ketosis while still making sure it has access to the vitamins, minerals, and other nutrients required to keep your body in good health.

The Best Autophagy-Inducing Diet

Designed to trigger a state of ketosis in which your body burns fat for energy instead of glucose, the keto diet is very strict about the ratio of macronutrients you consume.

75% of your calories should come from fat, 20% from protein, and only 5% from carbs.

There are variations of the keto diet, which are generally only used by bodybuilders or extreme athletes. The Targeted Keto Diet (TKD) adds carbs around workouts, and Cyclical versions include two days per week of higher-carb refeeds.

Finally, high protein versions use a ratio of 60:35:5 for fat:protein:carb.

Remember to work your way up to a high-fat, low-carb ratio in stages, and always keep in mind the quality of the food you're eating. Let's take a closer look at just what that might include. Or not.

What to Avoid

One of the reasons a lot of people turn towards a ketogenic diet is because of their belief that as long as they stay away from carbs, they can eat anything they want.

That might work to help you reach certain superficial goals, but it isn't right for the maintenance of good health.

There are quite a few foods, or food-like items, that you're going to want to avoid if you plan on making ketosis and autophagy a lifelong habit.

Though, most of the items on the avoid list are carbs. If you stay away from refined, highly processed carbohydrates, you will be reasonably successful at achieving ketosis. Some of the biggest keto offenders are:

- Refined and processed sugars like candy, soda, fruit juices, smoothies, and ice cream

- Grains and starches, especially refined versions such as bread, pasta, rice, and cereal

- Most fruit, especially dried fruits and very sweet fruits like bananas, apples, and figs

- Legumes, which include peas, beans, lentils, and chickpeas

- High-carb, starchy vegetables like roots and tubers, including beets, carrots, and potatoes

You're also going to want to stay away from low

fat or diet products, even if they're sugar-free or low-carb. Any time the food industry takes natural components out of food, they replace them with chemicals and additives that are no better for your health and, in many cases, are much worse.

You will also want to clear your fridge and cupboard of most pre-made condiments and sauces. These are almost always incredibly high in sugar, and even the smallest amount can sabotage an otherwise delicious and healthy keto-friendly meal.

There are even some fats that don't make the cut. Again, they are going to be highly processed options like vegetable oils and mayonnaise. They're too far from nature to provide any nourishment for your body and should not make it to your plate.

Finally, to follow a healthy ketogenic diet, you'll want to cut out alcohol. Spirits don't have any carbs, so technically they won't alter your ketosis if you drink them on the rocks, but there's evidence that drinking too much can inhibit autophagy, specifically in the liver. If you're socializing or celebrating, consider one glass of red wine. It's lower in carbs than beer, and it has the added benefit of polyphenol antioxidants, which are powerhouse nutrients.

There is a silver lining waiting for you still. In addition to avoiding certain foods, with a ketogenic diet, you can usually avoid counting calories.

When you first get started, it is a good idea to track what you're eating to make sure that you're consuming enough calories but not too many. Changing eating patterns will always confuse your body for a while, so it is helpful to have a way to track and measure. But once you're settled into a ketogenic plan, you shouldn't have to count or restrict calories.

When your body is healthy and being provided with high-quality nutrition, it will tell you when it's full. As long as you listen to it and stop eating when it sends the signal, you'll be self-regulating the number of calories you need.

When you eat a diet heavy in processed, fake foods and carbohydrates, you're much more likely to overeat. Your insulin response might be dysfunctional, and it's undoubtedly sending you mixed signals as your blood sugar levels continuously cycle through extreme highs and lows.

The other reason you may find yourself overeating is if you're malnourished. Nourishment is not measured exclusively by calories. Your body needs more than just energy from macronutrients to survive. It also requires micronutrients: vitamins and minerals.

If you eat a lot of processed food and not many nutrient-dense meals, your body will continue to demand that you feed it until it gets the nourishment that it needs.

In a whole-food-based ketogenic diet, you should easily be able to regulate your consumption without having to count calories.

What to Enjoy

Finally! You're going to learn what you can eat on a ketogenic diet.

Let's start by talking about healthy, natural fat sources.

- Meat, including red meat, pork, chicken, turkey

- Fatty fish like salmon, tuna, trout, mackerel

- Eggs, both the yolk and whites

- Full fat butter and cream

- Unprocessed cheese like goat, blue, mozzarella, cream or cheddar

- Nuts and seeds such as almonds, walnuts, flax, pumpkin, chia, etc.

- Healthy oils, meaning extra virgin olive oil, coconut, or avocado

- Avocados, coconuts, and olives themselves

Ideally, you'll want everything you eat to be organic and pasture-raised and finished. Since we're focusing on the autophagic benefits of a keto diet, we want to do our best not to reintroduce harmful chemicals and hormones that are found in factory-farmed meats and industrial agriculture.

People who don't understand a ketogenic diet might argue against it under the false assumption that because vegetables are considered carbs, you can't eat them and stay in ketosis. It is complete misinformation because there are plenty of vegetables that are amazingly high in nutritional value and low on the glycemic index. Some of the most beneficial vegetables for you to enjoy regularly include:

- Dark, leafy greens like Swiss chard, spinach, arugula, or romaine

- Cruciferous vegetables, including cabbage, kale, cauliflower, and broccoli, are low in carbs and extremely high in nutrition – many are even classified as superfoods

- Asparagus

- Certain nightshades, such as tomatoes, peppers, and eggplant but not potatoes

- Celery has very few carbs and plenty of nutrition, but the best part of it is that it is highly versatile. It makes a great snack – pile on the nut butter and munch away – as well as a perfect flavoring agent for cooked meals

There are so many vegetables and plants that it would be difficult to list them all here, but the above cover some of the most nutritionally dense and low-carb vegetables that are readily available in most areas of the world.

As you can see, as long as you avoid the highly starchy vegetables, you'll still have plenty of wonderful options to choose from to keep a fresh variety in your meal planning.

If you suffer from digestive issues or have the leaky gut syndrome and are using the ketogenic diet to try to heal and rebalance your gut flora, you may have trouble digesting some of these vegetables. If any of them are new to your eating plan, add them slowly, and see how your body reacts.

Fruits are just as controversial, as many people believe that because of their sugar content, they can't possibly be allowed within a keto diet. A lot of fruits are indeed going to be very hard on ketosis, but there are a few exceptions you can still eat to get the nutritional value of fruits.

Berries are the best fruit for you to reach for. They're full of potent antioxidants and delicious flavor. They're also quite small, so you can moderate your intake reasonably easily. Lemon does have a considerable amount of sugar in it, but you probably aren't going to eat enough lemon to destroy your ketosis efforts.

There are additional plant-based food items that can and should make it into your meal planning, namely natural herbs and spices. Since you'll be avoiding processed sauces and condiments, try adding flavor to your food using things like parsley, rosemary, or a little bit of garlic or ginger.

The antioxidants found in green and black tea are thought to support autophagy and cellular repair. One study discovered that the effects of green tea polyphenols have the power to mimic dietary restriction to induce a state of autophagy in your liver and also increased lipid, or fat, burning (Zhou et al., 2014). Essentially, it helps your body produce more AMPK, which triggers autophagy.

Another study found that this same autophagic flux would occur in kidneys that were damaged due to metabolic syndromes (Xie et al., 2017).

There have also been a few promising studies that suggest the anti-cancer benefits of ginger and turmeric may have some connection to autophagy. These are still relatively new areas of research, but adding these highly nutritious roots to your diet and fasting plan can't hurt.

The Discipline: Maintaining Autophagy

The most significant difference between dieting and choosing to change your lifestyle is that a diet has a specific end in mind, a goal to be finished.

A lifestyle, on the other hand, will last as long as you do.

Supporting autophagy in your body is more or less synonymous with supporting your health, and that is a lifestyle.

By following the eating and exercise plan outlined in this book, you'll not only be supporting the process of autophagy, but that, in turn, will help your metabolic system, which keeps you alive every single day.

Diets have a terrible reputation for not working in the long term because as soon as you stop and go back to your old habits, all your past grievances come back as well. When you find the discipline to maintain a lifestyle that supports autophagy, you'll be making lasting changes in your life. There's no reason to return to your old habits if you can enjoy and feel great with your habits.

Measuring Ketosis

When you're trying to improve your health through fitness or diet, it's essential to track your results. Enthusiasts track everything from the circumference of their waists and biceps to each morsel of food they've eaten and every physical movement taken.

Tracking your results is a fantastic motivational

tool to keep you progressing in the right direction, as well as to let you know if or when you fall off track.

There's another fundamental reason that tracking your momentum is a great way to ensure your success, and that has to do with bio-individuality. A diet that puts your spouse, friend, or a stranger into ketosis will not necessarily put you into ketosis.

Your unique body composition, daily movement, current metabolic functioning, and many more factors will force you to make small tweaks and changes to your diet and fasting schedule overtime to get the results you want. But the only way to know if you're truly succeeding is to track diligently.

It's surprisingly easy to track ketosis and predict how autophagy is operating within your own body.

You'll need only a few tools: a glucose meter, a ketone meter, and the strips required for testing your blood for each. You can check your blood once a day at the same time each day, or even multiple times a day if you'd like to track the changes as they happen.

After testing your blood, you can apply the Glucose Ketone Index (GKI) to decide whether you're in ketosis or not. To find your ratio, you simply divide your glucose levels – in millimoles – by your ketone levels, also in millimoles.

As mentioned in earlier chapters, anyone following a Standard American Diet (SAD) will likely have a ratio between 30 and 50. As you fast or get more acclimated to a ketogenic diet, the rate will get lower and lower.

Anything over 9 tells you that you still don't have enough ketones in your blood to have put you into a state of ketosis.

You'll start to see benefits from being in a ketotic state when the ratio dips below that magic number of 9, and the benefits will continue to become more noticeable the closer you get to a 1:1 ratio of glucose to ketones.

You could start to see weight loss or at least healthy weight maintenance, a reduction in Type 2 Diabetes, and noticeable improvements to brain damage or cognitive decline symptoms.

Most of the benefits achievable with a ratio between 3 and 9 are hormonal, related to insulin, and your metabolic system. In order to get the full therapeutic benefits of ketosis and autophagy, your ratio needs to be within the range of 1 or 2 (Ekberg, 2019).

The more in tune with your results you are, the better you'll be able to recognize the difference between metabolic benefits and autophagic benefits. Keep in mind, many of the benefits of autophagy are preventive and, therefore, harder to track or measure, unless you have a specific disease or disorder that you're trying to reverse.

Achieving and Maintaining Autophagy

Everything that you have learned so far should be approached and attempted with the utmost patience.

Trying to go from a Standard American Diet (SAD) and sedentary lifestyle to a 7-day water fast and daily HIIT fitness regime is not only dangerous to your immediate wellbeing, but it's likely also too extreme to be sustainable and have long-term benefits for you.

Choosing to improve your health is a life-long commitment. While we may use the word "diet" frequently, this is not meant to be a short-term fix or weight loss miracle cure. Whether you're starting in ill-health or relatively good health, it took you a lifetime to get where you are today, and you shouldn't expect to reverse damage overnight.

With that being said, you can work your way up to an optimal autophagic state through the following stages:

1. Reduce carbs in your diet. It should be your first step because it will help you regulate the extreme high and low blood sugar rollercoaster, and stabilize your energy levels overall. Reduce them slowly and healthfully, removing processed, nutrient-deficient carbs and increasing the quality of the carbs you do eat at the same time.

2. Start intermittent fasting. While there are many different types of fasting for you to choose from, merely decreasing your feeding window each day is one of the easiest ways to work fasting into your lifestyle. Start with at least 12 hours between your last meal of the day and the first meal of your next day. After a week, increase your fast to 13 hours. The week after that, make sure you only eat within a 10-hour window. Work your way up to a

16:8 schedule gradually and maintain that daily.

3. Increase your healthy fat consumption. Reducing carbs might naturally decrease your caloric intake, but you also want to be sure you're increasing the amount of fat you get in your diet, while still making sure you don't exceed a healthy level of calories. Focus on whole food fats like avocados, nuts, seeds, organic full-fat dairy and meats, and healthy, high-quality oils.

4. Commit to at least 20 minutes of HIIT training, three times a week or more.

5. Maintain your results through regular Intermittent Fasting (IF), exercise, and a low-carb or ketogenic eating plan.

6. Measure your Glucose Ketone Index (GKI) at least once a week.

7. Once you have some experience with fasting, try a longer water-fast. A 36-hour or 48-hour fast.

8. Cultivate other habits that are crucial to your overall health like getting enough sleep each night, and reducing daily stress.

Once you've found your unique sweet spot, you should feel energetic, satisfied, and healthy. Take a moment to appreciate this. Being healthy doesn't have to hurt to work.

Not everything beneficial for you must be painful or hard. It's often quite the opposite.

The harder a diet or exercise regimen is to maintain, the more you hate it, and the worse it hurts, the less likely you are to stick to it. You might see a few short-term perks, but in the long run, it will fail you.

If you take the time to work yourself up to healthy ketosis and establish balanced routines of exercise and fasting, you should thoroughly enjoy maintaining this new, healthy lifestyle.

The Fountain of Youth

D.R Krauz

Chapter 6:

Know When to Fold

There's a saying that goes, "All good things must come to an end."

You can indeed have too much autophagy taking place in your body, which might lead to side-effects: muscle loss, or dysregulated autophagy that starts to eat healthy cells or feed diseased cells.

For that to occur, you would most likely be abusing the techniques provided in this book. Exercising obsessively, fasting for too long, or eating unhealthy and nutrient-deficient foods, might take autophagy too far.

However, developing a safe and well-balanced, fasting, and ketogenic routine with regular exercise is a lifestyle change that can be adopted for life.

If you notice persistent side-effects, of course,

you'll want to consult with your doctor and find out what is wrong. There is no single diet or exercise program that is going to work for everyone.

A positive autophagy-inducing lifestyle, like the one I've outlined in this book, should be safe for most people to maintain for life. But you are the one to decide whether it works for you.

How Long Does Autophagy Take

We've discussed quite extensively how long it takes to induce autophagy in the body through different methods. The next question we need to ask is, how long do we need autophagy to be activated to produce noticeable results?

Just like every individual body is going to reach autophagy at different rates, every particular body is also going to have different levels of damage, toxins, and bacteria to cleanout.

As soon as autophagy begins, it will have some positive results. Each morsel of damaged material that is removed and recycled is one less worry for you.

A healthy person is going to have less damage to clean up than someone who is already suffering the effects of a disease or disorder.

The information in this book is not designed to help you induce autophagy once and then go on with your life, thinking you're cured and safe from all diseases.

Autophagy is a process of maintenance that needs to occur regularly to keep your body clean and healthy long-term.

The longer you spend in a fast, the longer your body will have to recycle old material at once. But a daily practice of intermittent fasting and staying in ketosis will keep autophagy active on a regular schedule.

Setting up a consistent schedule will not only keep your cells tidy at all times, but it also protects you from dysregulated autophagy, which can be harmful to your health. The idea that practice makes perfect applies well to the process of autophagy.

Even if you follow the suggestions in this book to the letter, there's no guarantee you'll see noticeable results at all. If you're already in reasonably good health, autophagy could be running in perfect order, and you may not notice at all.

The absence of symptoms is no guarantee that you're healthy, but it's also not a sign that something is wrong.

The benefits may also be so gradual that you don't notice them on a day to day basis. Something like insulin resistance is trackable, and you can pay attention to whether your response is improving and at what rate.

But cognitive function, on the other hand, can be much harder to compare. Do you have less brain fog today than yesterday? Was it due to autophagy or the fact that you got a great night's sleep? Was the good night's sleep a stroke of luck, or was it thanks to the process of autophagy?

Unless you're part of a scientific, clinical trial, there are too many variables at play to ever say definitively that specific results are the product of autophagy. It's also challenging to prove the opposite.

Pulling the Plug

Everything we know about health hinges on maintaining a very delicate balance. Human bodies are truly remarkable in their precision, and everything, from our pH to the composition of our total mass, needs to be kept at a perfect balance to operate effectively.

Your metabolic system does most of the balancing act for you, but how you eat, move, and rest your body impacts this delicate balance.

By this point in the book, I hope you're convinced of the benefits of inducing autophagy. However, you mustn't abuse the process and take it too far. You need to strike the right balance.

In the most extreme sense, even though fasting and exercise are healthy ways to kickstart your autophagy, if you stop eating altogether and never stop working your body, you will die.

The goal is to find a balance primarily between the anabolic and catabolic reactions, building up and breaking down all of the cells inside your body in a perfectly synced rhythm.

Historically, humans have been forced into cycles of feast and famine due to the difficulty of sourcing food. Their bodies were made to handle and thrive under these circumstances.

It's only in recent times that food has become so readily available that humans subsist in a constant phase of feasting.

Feeling hungry is your body's way of telling you that it's running low on easily accessible energy, and it's uncomfortable. It's not, however, life-threatening.

We don't like feeling uncomfortable, though, so if we feel a pang of hunger and food is available, we'll eat it and feel better at the moment. Feasting feeds anabolic reactions, but it reduces the need for catabolic reactions, disrupting the balance between them.

By using the techniques discussed in the last chapter, we can bring our bodies back into balance.

If you go too far, however, you can tip the scales in the opposite direction, which is just as unhealthy if sustained.

Ultimately, if you feel great practicing the habits in this book, there's no reason to stop. If you're experiencing side effects, you may need to take a break. The next chapter will go more in-depth on learning how to listen to your body, but ultimately you are the only one who can decide when it's time to pull the plug, if ever.

Staying Safe and Healthy

Autophagy is a very efficient and completely natural system that has some incredible benefits. As you'll find with most things in life, unfortunately, you can always have too much of a good thing.

What we know about autophagy is still limited, and every year this field is sure to advance with new and promising knowledge. What we do know, however, is that following a lifestyle that is scientifically proven to help the human body operate efficiently is going to help you enjoy more health throughout your lifetime.

It's impossible to predict lifespan. There are too many variables. However, you can influence the quality of life you have as you live out your natural lifespan. Autophagy is nature's way of keeping all the cells that make you who you are in optimal health for the longest time possible.

That is good news.

There is a point where too much autophagy – or too much fasting, fat, or exercise – can become harmful. If you deprive your body of protein for too long, you will be at risk for sarcopenia, which is loss of muscle mass and strength. Moreover, if you restrict your diet too much, you run the risk of eliminating vital vitamins, minerals, and antioxidants.

If you're underweight, have nutritional deficiencies, or if you have a history of disordered eating, fasting might not be the best option for your body.

If you are a very active person, you might have to adjust the fasting practices and the diet to meet your unique needs.

If you're pregnant, trying to get pregnant, or breastfeeding, long term fasting could leave you lacking in nutrients. Even Intermittent Fasting (IF) and ketosis should be approached with caution and your doctor's supervision.

Autophagy is one process by which your body keeps you healthy, and it's essential to keep your body in a condition that allows this process to take place when it needs to.

But that should never come at the detriment to the numerous other vital processes that are also working very hard to keep you healthy.

As you get older, you'll be in a position to need and benefit from autophagy even more, but the risks can be compounded, making you even more susceptible to muscle loss and frailty. Adjusting protein levels can help, but again, always be sure to get regular consultations with your primary care provider who can monitor your overall health.

We know some bacteria and parasites use autophagy to replicate themselves, and that in certain studies it appears autophagy increases the rate of cancer cell growth. Autophagy may also protect cancer cells from chemotherapy, making them harder to kill. If you have a bacterial infection or cancer, autophagy may not be right for you right now.

Whenever you begin any new health protocol, especially one that makes significant alterations to your diet or exercise practices, you must check in with your health practitioner first. It's also highly advisable that you make the changes slow and steady, and avoid taking any extreme measures all at once.

D.R Krauz

Chapter 7:

Autophagy for Life

Autophagy is not a one-time fix for all your health and wellness problems. It is going to take work and dedication and, once you find a great routine, it can be a life plan. Biological processes don't stop when you're healthy. They work hard every day of your life trying to keep you healthy.

You need to make sure that you're supporting all the biological processes inside your body, not just autophagy, every day. If you don't want your body to give up on you, you can't give up on your body.

Whenever you make significant changes to your lifestyle, you're bound to make a mistake here and there and possibly suffer some side effects because of it. Knowing ahead of time, what might go wrong will help you avoid making the most common mistakes.

If you can transition to an autophagic lifestyle relatively smoothly, and with the right mindset, there's no reason you can't keep it up for life.

Common Fasting & Ketosis Mistakes

The biggest mistake most people make when starting to fast and when transitioning to a high-fat diet is that they let themselves get dehydrated. Unless you're on a dry fast, make sure you're drinking plenty of water and keeping your electrolytes balanced.

You may even want to try supplementing sodium, potassium, and magnesium. You can get these minerals through a healthy keto diet, incorporating unrefined salt, spinach, and leafy greens, seeds, and avocados regularly.

As your insulin response is challenged and gradually balances out, your hydration will suffer. If you're not taking proactive steps to balance out the changes, you could experience dizziness, fatigue, headaches, and even dry mouth. Keeping yourself hydrated is an easy solution, and an excellent health hack on many levels.

The next most common mistake people make is not tracking what they're eating. Especially when you first start a ketogenic diet, it can be complicated to measure your servings of protein or carbs. It's easy to underestimate how many carbs you're eating, especially when you're used to a Standard American Diet (SAD). It's just as easy to overestimate how many fats you're eating, especially when you may still be harboring some fears that are difficult to leave behind.

Using a food tracker and having a kitchen scale is going to help you make sure you stick to your macros.

Similarly, getting yourself a glucose and ketone meter will help make sure that you're entering into ketosis. Eating a high-fat diet without getting into the optimal zone is selling yourself short. If this is a lifestyle change you plan on committing to for life, it's worth the investment to make sure you're doing it right.

And finally, another common mistake that some people make when they approach either fasting or keto is using it as an excuse to eat garbage. Once again, it's vital that you understand the difference between weight loss and health.

Even if it's possible to lose weight eating high-fat, low-carb junk food while fasting, that doesn't make it healthy. Triggering your body's natural defense against internal cellular damage is going to be completely negated if you're not providing your body with the highest quality of nutrition that you can manage while you follow the process.

Mindset

Being able to stick to any new habits or lifestyle change is often more about your mindset than it is about the change itself.

Truly understanding why you're committing to these autophagy-inducing processes is going to be what saves you from caving in to cravings, or giving up when things get tough.

There will be moments when you don't want to do this anymore. Remembering why you started in the first place, as long as your reasons are powerful, they'll keep you going for the long run.

It's also important not to let exercise, fasting, ketosis, or your fascination with autophagy rule your life. When you begin making changes in your life to support autophagy, some of the practices may seem extreme compared to your current comfort zone.

It will get easier, and you'll get used to it over time, but while you're transitioning, you don't want to let obsession take over. You are still human, and you don't have to follow every piece of advice to the letter every single day for the rest of your life. If you mess up, it won't kill you.

Be patient and forgiving with yourself.

And finally, keep reminding yourself that you didn't get into the condition you're in right now overnight. You shouldn't expect to see dramatic changes overnight, either.

The results will come, and you will start to feel fantastic every day.

When that happens, don't stop what's working. Don't fall back into unhealthy habits when you reach your goals.

Understanding and Listening To Your Body

A well-functioning and healthy body will send signals to help you understand what it needs to survive. That's why you frequently hear experts telling you to "listen to your body."

Unfortunately, our modern lifestyle has forced our bodies to lie to us and mislead us.

Not only that, but it's important to remember that the absence of symptoms of sickness or disease is not the same as health. Illness and disease can sometimes take days, weeks, or even years to show their signs, but that doesn't mean they don't exist in your body.

If you wait until you see symptoms until your body screams at you that something's wrong, you'll already be too late in some cases, and in most others, you'll at the very least already be at a disadvantage.

Proactively maintaining health to prevent disease is much easier than reactively trying to treat and cure it. As you know, many disorders don't have known cures, and many others have treatment processes that are brutal and come with a wide variety of side effects.

I hope you'll agree that it's much preferable to not get sick in the first place.

Glucose has been discussed in every single chapter of this book because it has such overarching impacts on our health and how our entire body operates. Yes, it impacts the functioning of autophagy, but it goes much beyond that single process.

Sugar is addicting, especially when it's highly refined and devoid of the natural vitamins, minerals, and fiber that accompany glucose in a whole food source like an apple. Some studies even suggest that refined sugar is more addictive than cocaine.

It alters the way your body communicates with you. When you're addicted to any substance, your body will start sending signals to convince you that you need more of that substance, not because it's critical to your survival, but because of the chemical addiction.

So if you're reading this book, get ready to follow the instructions for transitioning from a Standard American Diet (SAD) to a low-carb or ketogenic diet boosted by intermittent fasting. Not only will you need to adapt your body to the new cycle of feeding, but you'll also likely be going through symptoms of withdrawal and detoxification.

What to Expect

Understanding what's happening inside your body as you progress will help you decipher the signals your body is giving you, learning when you genuinely need specific sustenance for your health and survival, and when your body is lying to you.

A lot of this process will come down to common sense. If your body starts telling you that it is in desperate need of a slice of chocolate cake, but it has absolutely no interest in a banana, it's probably lying to you.

Fat and protein are much more satiating than carbs, so your cravings aren't likely to come from hunger, but most people are addicted to sugar. You should expect to experience cravings for sugar, even if you never thought you had a sweet-tooth. You may think you eliminated bread and pasta, but all your body knows is that it's not getting its sugar fix.

Where things will become more complicated is when you start to feel drained of energy. You might wonder if it's because your body is adjusting to your new regimen and needs a little more time to adapt, or if you're truly in a danger zone.

In terms of fasting, it's usually safer to err on the side of caution. Start by making sure you're hydrated and are getting enough electrolytes, but if symptoms still progress, you might want to break your fast with whole food, keto-friendly options, and try again on another day.

If it's the ketogenic diet that's causing you to feel

brain fog or cramping, try altering the type of food options you're choosing, rather than the macronutrients themselves. You might have a sensitivity to a particular food, which is common with dairy, eggs, and even some vegetables. If you're overcoming digestive issues like leaky gut, consulting a registered dietician might help get you adjusted.

Those who jump straight into the ketogenic diet without taking the time to gradually get their digestive system used to the new order of things sometimes report catching "the keto flu."

Symptoms are similar to what you would experience with common flu, namely fatigue, stomach pain, and dizziness, to varying degrees.

It happens because you are ingesting much more fat that your body is used to, and it doesn't know what to do with it all. For others, it's more of a response to carbohydrate restriction and is similar to what you would go through if you were coming out of an addiction. Either way, making the process slow and steady should save you from the worst of these side effects.

Detoxifying

Part of getting healthier is removing unhealthy components from inside your body. That's precisely why we want to trigger autophagy, after all.

But where autophagy recycles the waste and damaged materials, detoxifying is simply a process of removing it from your body.

It happens naturally every day. Through sweat, what we leave in the bathroom, and even a sneeze, our body has its ways of getting toxic materials out.

When you fast, exercise, or start a healthy new diet, part of healing will be detoxifying, with or without autophagy.

And detox can be unpleasant.

If you follow the advice of working your way up to longer fasts and full ketosis gradually, the detoxifying process will also be gradual, and hopefully not too noticeable.

If you shock your system, however, you may find yourself experiencing symptoms similar to going through withdrawal: headaches, mood swings, trouble sleeping, or feeling entirely wakeful, aches, and pains.

Many people experience breakouts as toxic materials are expelled through your pores. Digestive issues are normal as your body gets used to new foods and eating patterns.

If you expect to experience these symptoms, you won't be wholly disillusioned with the program if they occur. If you don't experience them, you can revel in the fact that your body adapts quickly.

If any of the symptoms last for longer than a few days or feel extreme, stop the program. Consult your doctor. Try again more slowly.

There are ways to lessen or avoid the symptoms altogether.

First and foremost, you want to make sure you're always well hydrated. It will not only help you feel satiated and train your body to understand the difference between hunger and thirst, but it's also one of the main ways your body flushes out toxins.

You'll also want to regulate your fiber intake. If you're eating more plant-based foods than you're used to, you may find yourself a bit constipated as you get used to the fiber. On the other hand, if you cut back on the fruits and vegetables you're used to eating to eliminate carbs and sugars, you might find yourself lacking in fiber.

Everyone is going to react slightly differently, but your body will adjust.

Sweating is a great way to get toxins out of your system, so don't shirk the exercise portion of this program even if the fasting and new diet seem to be enough to help you see results. Exercise is critical for overall health.

Finally, you'll want to make sure you get plenty of rest. Eight hours every night, ideally for the rest of your life, and maybe even more while you're fasting. Remember, this is the best time for your body to heal, and that includes dealing with toxins.

Advocate for Yourself

Once upon a time, people didn't have specialized doctors, nutritionists, and personal trainers to tell us how to take care of our bodies. But over the past century or so, we've started listening to what other people tell us about what is right for our bodies, and we've individually lost the ability to recognize for ourselves what makes us feel great.

Every other animal on earth eats intuitively to survive and thrive. Every other animal exists healthfully on natural ingredients.

Because humans can create food-like options and enhance what occurs naturally, we do. We can grow food larger, faster, and sweeter through chemicals, hormones, and other additives, so we do. We've learned how to protect our food from other creatures who want to eat it through the use of pesticides and herbicides, so we do.

All of these actions make food easier to produce and cheaper in some ways, and therefore we consider these processes better. But faster, cheaper, and more plentiful does not equal more healthful.

We've also accepted a state of being that believes some level of discomfort is normal or natural.

You've had constipation issues for years; it must be normal.

You haven't been able to get a good night's sleep since you were in your teens. It must be normal.

You can't lose weight; it must be hormones, or hereditary, or simply your cross to bear in life.

None of those statements are true.

Normal, in comparison to an increasingly sick population, isn't a great yardstick to measure by.

Human bodies are made to be healthy and strong. If something is making you uncomfortable and ill, it's up to you to decide it isn't natural or normal. You don't have to live in pain.

One of the most effective ways to heal your body and relearn how to listen to it is to return to eating as many whole and natural foods as possible. Avoid processed foods with a lot of additives, and you'll automatically be headed in the right direction.

Eat when you're hungry and stop eating when you're full. Know the difference between dehydration and hunger. Find ways to comfort and destress and enjoy your life that doesn't include putting yourself into a food coma.

Pay attention to savoring the food you eat, rather than rushing to eat as much as you possibly can.

Your body is an incredibly complex machine with systems and components that we still don't understand completely. But it is surprisingly simple to keep it maintained when you give it what it needs to survive.

Autophagy and ketosis will help bring a struggling body back to proper working order and can be a life-long lifestyle change that keeps your body running healthfully.

The Fountain of Youth

D.R Krauz

Conclusion

This book may or may not be the map to the exact location of the mythical Fountain of Youth. That's something only you can find out with time. Still, it has provided you with valuable insights into how you can activate the self-healing properties of autophagy.

Your cells are being damaged with every breath you take and every move you make. Still, your body is designed to heal that damage in the most efficient way possible: by removing useless cellular material and recycling it into energy that can be used to heal, protect, and defend your healthy cells.

Just like any powerful machine, your body needs to be maintained regularly to run smoothly and efficiently — autophagy to the rescue.

Be In The Know

When a single biological process is the leading factor behind two separate Nobel Prizes, barely 40 years apart, it's a pretty good indicator that the research is life-changing.

Thanks to Christian de Duve, the existence and basic operations of autophagy were discovered, and Yoshinori Ohsumi built upon this knowledge to identify the functions and mechanisms of the process. Because Ohsumi believed that the process of cell degradation deserved just as much attention as synthesis, we now have a basic understanding of how cells can withstand malnourishment, infections, and even some diseases.

Cells have a hard life. To keep up with the demand for operating an entire human body every single day, they must not only have a way to heal themselves, but they have to be very efficient at finding and tapping a reliable power source.

Your digestive system uses a variety of acids and enzymes to take what you eat and disassemble it so that it can be absorbed and used by our bodies. Your metabolic system determines how that energy gets put to use - either building, in an anabolic reaction, or in demolishing, which is a catabolic reaction.

Above all, your body appreciates balance, so these systems have to have their communication just right to make sure our bodies get what they need.

By keeping the playing field clean and tidy, and all the equipment in good repair, autophagy helps make sure operations run as they should.

Autophagy can rescue and heal damaged cells, or it can destroy them and use them for parts. Stress, bacteria and viruses, environmental pollutants, and especially what we eat all cause damage and unwelcome build-up inside our cells. Just because we can't see it doesn't mean it's not potentially life-threatening.

Scientific studies have watched and marveled at the process of autophagy working to prevent disease, keeping cells young, healthy, and strong, and also protecting our brain in many ways.

Just by adapting to a few lifestyle changes, changes that arguably better reflect how humans were designed to live in the first place, we can give our bodies the time and nutrition they require to keep this process of autophagy working optimally.

Modern science and medicine are truly impressive and have discovered many ways to treat and sometimes even eradicate symptoms of many diseases. But wouldn't it be nice to not get sick in the first place?

Life in the 21st century is a lot more comfortable

than it was 100 years ago; there's no doubt about that. But it many ways, it's also hurting us and decreasing our quality of life.

Human beings may now live longer lives than they had the opportunity to do historically, but we're also collectively spending more years sick and damaged.

Living a long life is a beautiful dream, but it loses a lot of its luster if the last 10, 20, or even 30 years of your life are spent suffering. It doesn't have to be that way.

We've learned so much that we know it's possible to become a healthy, vibrant centenarian with continued strong mental capacity. If it's possible, it should be our goal.

The power of autophagy makes that goal attainable.

Of course, it isn't a miracle cure or pill for instant health. It requires constant dedication, and there's no guarantee that you will be wholly protected from sickness and disease.

If you're willing to put in the effort to treat your body well, the results will be worth it.

Reversing years' worth of damage, even though a

gentle and natural process like autophagy, won't be without its difficulties.

Exercise is hard - physically, mentally, and emotionally, especially if it's new to your daily practice. But every time you do it, you will get stronger and more powerful. Your body was made to move. It craves it and needs it to survive. Your brain might tell you otherwise at first, but it will also benefit from exercise in many ways. After a while, even your brain will crave the activity. It will get easier.

Fasting is hard - especially if you're used to free-feeding whenever the urge takes you. You are not alone. A growing number of people in the world are using food not as energy for their body, but as comfort, entertainment, and escape. If you find those things outside of food, feeding your body to fuel it will become easier. Fasting will get easier. And your body will adapt, making it easier and helping you get stronger and more resistant to stress in the process.

Ironically, following a keto diet for most people is the easiest element of the autophagic lifestyle, but it can mentally be the most difficult. We've been programmed by society to look at fat with terror, that it's hard to let go of the fear. Education and personal experience will become your most significant defenses here.

The cells in your body are designed to use either glucose or ketones for fuel. The first is easy but leads to serious blood sugar issues. The second is a bit more work for your body, but it keeps hormones balanced, your brain healthy, and, it turns out, a bit more work is good for quality control.

If you stick to a lifestyle designed to support a healthy autophagic process and give your body time to heal, it will get easier every day. You will feel healthier because your body will be running more efficiently. And once you start feeling the real effects of health, you won't ever want to go back to feeling the effects of disease.

Action Is More Powerful Than Knowledge

Reading this book and doing some additional research on the subject of autophagy is a significant first step. But you could be the world's foremost expert on autophagy, and If you are not taking daily action to support it, all the knowledge and understanding in the world isn't going to do anything for your health.

You need to start making real changes if you want

to see a real difference in your health. It's time to put the principles of autophagy into practice in your own life.

You must take your time and adapt your body to the changes gradually. Start where you are. Don't base your progress on anything but your results. Aim to get a little more effective each day.

Above all, remember that all bodies react to exercise, fasting, and ketosis differently. Listening to your own body is the only way you will be able to find out what works for you. Comparing yourself to others is never ideal, but even more so in this situation.

What one person does to see results will not necessarily be what you need to do. Age, gender, and size are the simplest variables that make significant differences to results. But your current state of insulin sensitivity, how many toxins your body is holding onto, how much muscle mass you have, and how much build-up there is on your heart and brain when you start the process - all these factors will affect your practice. They're much more difficult to see.

That's why listening to your own body and having patience are crucial to your overall success.

Even if you can reach some or many of your goals through diet alone, exercise is still a vital component of a healthy, autophagy-inducing lifestyle. Do not skip this step.

Depending on your current capabilities, you may need to start by simply adding a 20-minute walk to your day. If that's easy, try jogging instead. If that's no problem, add some interval sprints in there.

Work your way up to a HIIT program safely and, ideally, with the help of a professional who can monitor your heart rate to help keep you safe and also so you can watch yourself improve.

HIIT is the most effective way to see tangible results in both cardiovascular measures as well as strength and muscle building. But perhaps more importantly, it's also one of the best ways to safely induce autophagy without adding more damage to your body in the process.

Intermittent fasting will not only improve your efforts with exercise, but it will also keep autophagy working hard for you. Again, it's important to start where you are and change your eating habits safely.

If you're used to eating every 2 hours and you

decide to try a 3-day water-fast, you are not doing yourself any favors. Any time you search for a one-time, quick fix, you're more likely to give up before seeing lasting results.

Instead, gradually start decreasing your feeding window each day. Start slow. As your body learns to trust you, progress will get faster. For most people, the jump from 10 hours of fasting to 11 hours is much harder than the increase from 15 to 16. Trust the process, and don't give up.

Fasting is one of the best ways you can naturally induce autophagy. When your cells don't have a consistent supply of easy energy, they will go hunting for other options. Instead of adding more chemicals and additives to the debris accumulating in your body, and instead of causing yet another spike and subsequent crash of blood glucose, autophagy can recycle all the leftovers causing troubles in your cells already.

To practice Intermittent Fasting (IF) regularly has been shown to help you live longer and improve the quality of your life at the same time. Age gracefully and with dignity, keep your body strong and active, and your brain functioning at full capacity.

As a bonus, with fewer meals to worry about,

you'll be saving yourself time and money to devote to enjoying your life in other, more meaningful ways.

Fasting and starvation are different things don't forget, so when you are feeding, make sure the quality of the food is the best you can afford. It's so important to make sure you are nourished as well as energized.

We know that autophagy will start working inside your cells much quicker if you're in a state of ketosis, so following a healthy keto diet will help you maintain the most effective autophagic lifestyle overall.

70% of your daily calories should be coming from high-quality fats. Look for organic meats, fatty fish, eggs, and dairy products. Incorporate also plant-based fat sources like nuts, seeds, avocado, and certain oils. Stay away from highly processed foods. Not all fat is made equal.

25% of your diet should be high-quality protein, a lot of which will be accounted for already, just by eating the foods listed above. Animal products, as well as nuts and seeds, are all excellent sources of protein.

Finally, limit your carbohydrate intake to only 5%

of your daily calories, and make them count. A slice of bread might be enticing, but it's not going to provide you with anything but a guilty pleasure. Instead, look for low-carb, high nutritional value vegetables, like cauliflower, leafy greens, and tomatoes or cucumber.

Don't forget that you need micronutrients as much as you need macronutrients. Most of your vitamins and minerals are going to come from bright, colorful vegetables, so you must choose your carbs wisely.

Aside from helping to induce autophagy, following a keto diet has been shown to have incredible neuroprotective benefits, as well as to help manage diabetes and other insulin-related disorders such as weight gain, heart disease, and PCOS.

If you make these changes slowly and consistently, it should be relatively easy and enjoyable to maintain this lifestyle long term.

It's a good idea to track and measure your process to make sure that you're actually getting into ketosis and the ideal GKI to induce autophagy. Following these habits will help your body get healthier in many ways, but the overall purpose is to make sure you're getting the full benefits and healing power of autophagy.

Once you know you're effectively utilizing exercise, fasting, and ketosis, all you have to do is find your rhythm and enjoy the results!

Be Smart, Stay Safe

Above all, when you're making any significant lifestyle changes like the ones suggested in this book, you must stay safe. It's easy to become obsessed and get caught up in grandiose plans, and that can cause more damage than it heals.

Autophagy is a highly individualized process. How long it takes to get started is different for everyone. How much work it has to accomplish is just as unique.

The more practiced you get at all of the autophagy inducing techniques, the more efficient your body will become at calling the clean-up crew. But it will take time.

It's been mentioned multiple times already, but autophagy is not a one-time quick fix. It should happen in your body regularly, for your entire life, which means you should be supporting it continually, for the rest of your life.

Having the right mindset from the start is going to help you maintain your results.

If you're looking for a quick, easy win, autophagy may not be for you. But if you want to live a healthy life, for the rest of your life, you will have to set your priorities accordingly.

There are short-term pleasures in life, like chasing a bucket of fried chicken with a 6-pack of beer.

And there are long-term pleasures, like learning how to tango when you're 60 years old, or hiking every weekend with your friends or family, or teaching your kids how to play sports by actually playing with them.

Short-term pleasures have consequences like weight gain, heartburn, lethargy, and the potential to develop several entirely preventable diseases.

Long-term pleasures have consequences like excitement and adventure, love and connection, pride and ambition.

You know which choice will give you the highest overall enjoyment out of life. The question simply comes down to whether or not you can make the rest of your life your priority at the cost of the next

5 minutes, or if you will decide to prioritize the next 5 minutes at the expense of the rest of your life.

Autophagy prioritizes your life.

Of course, with all that being said, some exercises, fasting protocols, and dietary plans will not work for everyone. If you consistently experience uncomfortable side-effects, you might have to tweak the strategy to suit you better.

You should always make any significant changes only after consulting with a doctor, especially if you currently have any health concerns.

Do your due diligence, though, and this includes finding a doctor that can understand and is willing to work with your goals. Just because you've had the same doctor for the last ten years doesn't mean he or she is the right choice for the next decade.

Integrative physicians who incorporate natural, holistic lifestyle changes into their traditional, allopathic methods are becoming more popular and might be a helpful resource for you as you work towards an autophagy-supporting lifestyle.

Do your diligence when it comes to applying the principles of exercise, fasting, and ketosis to your life as well. Find a support system or a mentor who can help guide you through the process in a way that will work best for you.

Learn from the mistakes others have already made so that you can transition as smoothly as possible. Know what to expect. All change is going to take time to get used to, and more often than not, the road to health is paved with minor discomfort. Know what's normal and will pass, and what might be a cause for concern.

Don't be scared to ask questions or for help. Trying to be the healthiest version of yourself is inspiring, and people will want to help you along the way. Let them.

Share your experiences with people you trust and who can support you, giving you the strength of mind to continue towards your goals, even when things get tough.

Changing your life is an individual decision, and you shouldn't expect anyone else to want to follow in your footsteps. Being open with your experiences and enthusiastic about your successes might encourage your loved ones to join you in becoming healthier themselves, and that is wonderful.

But the only person you can change is yourself. And the only person who should ever be responsible for your health is you.

Everyone needs to come to this decision for themselves, and the best thing you can do for your loved ones is to lead by example.

The healthier you get, and the more enjoyment out of life you start to feel, the more devoted you will become to this new lifestyle.

It may seem like a lot to take in right now, but it all starts with one small step in the right direction.

What will your next step be?

The Autophagy Lifestyle Planner

(<u>DO NOT</u> start this new life-path without a well-structured plan...)

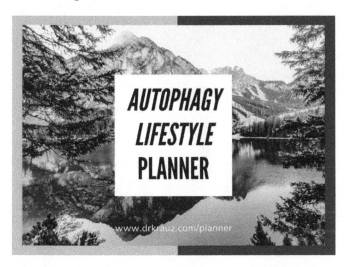

With the *Autophagy Lifestyle* Planner, you'll get:

> ➢ The **9 key elements** you cannot induce autophagy without.
> ➢ How to schedule them into your week, for maximum results.
> ➢ An effective way of keeping yourself accountable.

If you haven't done so, get your *Autophagy Lifestyle Planner,* right now:

www.drkrauz.com/planner

D.R Krauz

References

Autophagy. (2019). In Mirriam-Webster.com.

Retrieved August 19, 2019, from https://www.merriam-webster.com/medical/autophagy

Brigham Young University. (2017, May 10). High levels of exercise linked to nine years of less aging at the cellular level: New research shows a major advantage for those who are highly active. ScienceDaily. Retrieved August 24, 2019, from www.sciencedaily.com/releases/2017/05/170510115211.htm

CDC. (2017). Diet/Nutrition. Retrieved from https://www.cdc.gov/nchs/fastats/diet.htm

Chun, S.K., Lee, S., Yang, M.-J, Leeuwenburgh, C., Kim, J.-S, (2017). Exercise-Induced Autophagy in Fatty Liver Disease [PDF File]. Exercise and Sport Sciences Reviews, 45(3), 181–186. Retrieved from https://journals.lww.com/acsm-essr/FullText/2017/07000/Exercise_Induced_Autophagy_in_

Fatty_Liver_Disease.9.aspx#pdf-link

Dr.Education - FITNESS & NUTRITION. (2019). Unknown TRUTH about AUTOPHAGY | Dr. Education (Eng) [Video File]. Retrieved from https://youtu.be/_enmj_zAoHM

Ekberg, Dr. Sten [Dr. Sten Ekberg]. (2019, May 22). What Breaks a Fast? (True Fast vs. Intermittent Fasting) [Video File]. Retrieved from https://youtu.be/RGHOF8JfZ5g

Ekberg, Dr. Sten [Dr. Sten Ekberg]. (2019, July 8). Autophagy & Fasting: How Long To Biohack Your Body For Maximum Health? (GKI) [Video File]. Retrieved from https://youtu.be/96dv7Xrgksw

Galluzzi, L., Pietrocola, F., Bravo-San Pedro, J.-M., Amaravadi, R. K., Baehrecke, E. H., Cecconi, F., & ... Kroemer, G. (2015). Autophagy in malignant transformation and cancer progression. The Embo Journal, (34)7, 856-880. Doi: 10.15252/embj.201490784. Retrieved from https://www.ncbi.nlm.nih.gov/pmc/articles/PMC4388596/

Goldhammer, A., Lisle, D., Parpia, B., Anderson, S. V., & Campbell, T. C. (2001). Medically supervised water-only fasting in the treatment of hypertension. Journal of Manipulative and Physiological Therapeutics. 24(5). 335-339. Retrieved from https://doi.org/10.1067/mmt.2001.115263

Gonzalez, C. D., Alvarez, S., Ropolo, A., Rosenzvit, C., Gonzalez Bagnes, M. F., Vaccaro, M. I. (2014). Autophagy, Warburg, and Warburg Reverse Effects in Human Cancer. BioMed Research International, 2014. 10 pages. Retrieved from https://doi.org/10.1155/2014/926729

He, C., Bassik, M., Moresi, V., Sun, K., Wei, Y., Zou, Z., & ... Levine, B. (2012). Exercise-induced BCL2-regulated autophagy is required for muscle glucose homeostasis. Nature 481, 511–515. Retrieved from https://www.nature.com/articles/nature10758

Hutchinson, P. (n.d.), How Many Calories a Day Does the Average Body Burn? Retrieved August 24, 2019 from https://www.livestrong.com/article/315121-how-many-calories-a-day-does-the-average-body-burn/

Krebs, J. D., Parry Strong, A., Cresswell, P., Reynolds, A. N., Hanna, A., & Haeusler, S. (2016). A randomised trial of the feasibility of a low carbohydrate diet vs standard carbohydrate counting in adults with type 1 diabetes taking body weight into account [PDF file]. Asia Pac J Clin Nutr 25(1). 78-84. Retrieved from, http://apjcn.nhri.org.tw/server/APJCN/25/1/78.pdf

Land, Siim (2019, January 29). Autophagy and Exercise [Web log post]. Retrieved from http://siimland.com/autophagy-and-exercise/

Leow, Z. Z. X., Guelfi, K. J., Davis, E. A., Jones, T. W., Fournier, P. A. (2018, September). The glycaemic benefits of a very-low-carbohydrate ketogenic diet in adults with Type 1 diabetes mellitus may be opposed by increased hypoglycaemia risk and dyslipidaemia. Diabetic Medicine, 35(9), 1258-1263. Retrieved from, https://doi.org/10.1111/dme.13663

Mandal, A. (2019, February 26). History of the Ketogenic Diet. Retrieved on August 23, 2019 from https://www.news-medical.net/health/History-of-the-Ketogenic-Diet.aspx

Meidenbauer, J., Mukherjee, P. & Seyfried, T.N. (2015). The glucose ketone index calculator: A simple tool to monitor therapeutic efficacy for metabolic management of brain cancer. Nutrition & metabolism. 12(1). DOI: 10.1186/s12986-015-

0009-2. Retrieved from

https://www.researchgate.net/publication/2740
11072_The_glucose_ketone_index_calculator_
A_simple_tool_to_monitor_therapeutic_efficac
y_for_metabolic_management_of_brain_cance
r

Nobel Media AB. (2019) Otto Warburg. Retrieved
August 21, 2019 from
https://www.nobelprize.org/prizes/medicine/19
31/warburg/facts/

Nobel Media AB. (2019). The Nobel Prize in
Physiology or Medicine 1974. Retrieved August
19, 2019 from
https://www.nobelprize.org/prizes/medicine/19
74/summary/

Nobel Media AB. (2019). The Nobel Prize in
Physiology or Medicine 2016. Retrieved August
19, 2019 from
https://www.nobelprize.org/prizes/medicine/20
16/summary/

Takagi, A., Kume, S., Kondo, M., Nakazawa, J.,
Chin-Kanasaki, M., Araki, H., ... & Uzu, T. (2016,
January 06) Mammalian autophagy is essential
for hepatic and renal ketogenesis during
starvation. Sci. Rep. 6, 18944; doi:

10.1038/srep18944 (2016).

TEDx Talks. (2014, March 18). Why fasting bolsters brain power: Mark Mattson at TEDxJohnsHopkinsUniversity [Video file]. Retrieved from https://youtu.be/4UkZAwKoCP8

USDA. (2015). Dietary Guidelines for Americans 2015-2020 Eighth Edition [PDF]. Retrieved August 24, 2019, from https://health.gov/dietaryguidelines/2015/reso urces/2015-2020_Dietary_Guidelines.pdf

Whittel, N. [Naomi Whittel]. (2019, April 20). Rare Interview with Nobel Prize Winner, Dr. Yoshinori Ohsumi on Autophagy [Video file]. Retrieved from https://youtu.be/2O_r-d-HrjA

Whittel, N. [Naomi Whittel]. (2019, May 13). Autophagy 101 - Everything You Need to Know - with Dr. William Dunn [Video file]. Retrieved from https://youtu.be/ERKmJK_atdc

Whittel, N. [Naomi Whittel]. (2019, June 1). How to Activate Autophagy - TIPS with Christiaan Leeuwenburgh, PhD [Video file]. Retrieved from https://youtu.be/82cR8tqe6aw

Web of Stories - Life Stories of Remarkable People. (2017). Christian de Duve - Autophage: Self-eating by cells (45/106) [Video file].

Retrieved from https://youtu.be/8WXICTVS4jA

World Health Organization. (2018). Obesity and overweight. Retrieved August 24, 2019, from https://www.who.int/news-room/fact-sheets/detail/obesity-and-overweight#targetText=Of%20these%20over%20650%20million,tripled%20between%201975%20and%202016.

Xie, X., Yi, W., Zhang, P., Wu, N., Yan, Q., Yang, H., ... & Ying, C. (2017, May). Green Tea Polyphenols, Mimicking the Effects of Dietary Restriction, Ameliorate High-Fat Diet-Induced Kidney Injury via Regulating Autophagy Flux. Nutrients.9(5). 497. doi: 10.3390/nu9050497 Retrieved from, https://www.ncbi.nlm.nih.gov/pmc/articles/PMC5452227/

Zhou, J., Farah, B. L., Sinha, R. A., Wu, Y., Bay, B. H., ... & Yen, P. M. (2014, January 29). Epigallocatechin-3-gallate (EGCG), a green tea polyphenol, stimulates hepatic autophagy and lipid clearance. PLoS One. 9(1). doi: 10.1371/journal.pone.0087161 Retrieved from https://www.ncbi.nlm.nih.gov/pubmed/24489859

D.R Krauz

CPSIA information can be obtained
at www.ICGtesting.com
Printed in the USA
LVHW090533231219
641436LV00001B/178/P